CIRCADIAN DIET COOKBOOK FOR BEGINNERS

Enhance Metabolic Health, Weight Management, Hormone Optimization, Inflammation Reduction, Sleep Quality Enhancement, and Overall Well-being

Audrey McAllister, MD

Copyright PAGE

Requests for permission to use or reproduce any part of this publication should be addressed to the publisher in writing. The publisher reserves the right to grant or deny permission at their discretion, taking into consideration factors such as the intended use, nature of the excerpt, and potential impact on the original work.

Unauthorized reproduction or distribution of copyrighted material is a violation of intellectual property rights and may result in legal consequences. Individuals or entities found to be in breach of copyright law may be subject to legal action, including but not limited to injunctions, damages, and legal fees.

It is the responsibility of all users of this publication to familiarize themselves with and abide by copyright laws and regulations. By accessing or using any part of this work, individuals agree to comply with the terms and conditions set forth by the publisher regarding copyright protection and usage rights.

Table of Contents

SECTION 1: THE CIRCADIAN DIET

The fundamental principle underlying the Circadian Diet revolves around the synchronization of eating habits with the body's intrinsic 24-hour clock, which governs a myriad of physiological processes. This dietary approach acknowledges the dynamic nature of the body's metabolic and hormonal fluctuations throughout the day, suggesting that aligning meal times with these natural cycles can promote overall health and well-being.

Central to the Circadian Diet is the concept of Time-Restricted Eating (TRE), wherein individuals restrict the window of time during which food can be consumed. This often involves adhering to a structured eating schedule characterized by a fasting period lasting 12–16 hours, followed by designated eating hours. The rationale behind TRE is rooted in the belief that the body's metabolism operates optimally during specific periods, thereby advocating for strategic meal timing to enhance metabolic efficiency.

Equally important in the Circadian Diet is the timing of meals, with proponents recommending heartier breakfasts and lighter evening meals. This approach aligns with the body's natural metabolic rhythm, as metabolism tends to peak during waking hours, necessitating greater energy intake earlier in the day.

Nutritional timing also plays a significant role, emphasizing the importance of consuming certain nutrients at specific times of the day. For instance, carbohydrates and protein may be prioritized earlier in the day to fuel energy needs, while healthy fats are favored in the evening to support satiety and promote restorative processes during sleep. The overarching objective is to optimize nutrient intake in a manner that complements the body's circadian cycle and supports metabolic function.

In essence, the Circadian Diet embodies an integrative approach to nutrition, emphasizing harmony with the body's natural circadian rhythm. Proponents of this dietary philosophy aspire to enhance metabolic function, boost energy levels, and promote overall health by incorporating principles of Time-Restricted Eating, meal timing, and nutritional optimization. While research in this area continues to evolve, there is growing evidence suggesting that aligning eating habits with circadian rhythms may confer various health benefits. However, individual responses to such dietary interventions may vary, highlighting the need for personalized approaches to optimize outcomes.

The influence of natural cycles on well-being

The intrinsic connection between rhythms and health underscores the intricate interplay of biological processes within the human body. Among these rhythms, the 24-hour circadian cycle stands out as paramount, orchestrating a myriad of physiological and behavioral functions. It is the synchronization of this internal clock with external cues, primarily the natural light-dark cycle, that maintains harmony between our internal rhythm and the surrounding environment.

Circadian rhythms exert profound influence over metabolism, hormone secretion, temperature regulation, and the sleep-wake cycle. Disruption of this rhythm, whether due to shift work, jet lag, or irregular sleep patterns, can significantly compromise health. Research indicates that circadian misalignment may lead to a spectrum of health issues, including sleep disorders, metabolic disturbances, psychological ailments, and heightened susceptibility to chronic diseases like diabetes and cardiovascular conditions.

Beyond the circadian rhythm, numerous other biological cycles impact health. Ultradian rhythms, occurring within a 24-hour span, regulate shorter cycles such as hormone pulses and periods of alertness and rest. Conversely, infradian rhythms, exemplified by the menstrual cycle in females, extend beyond the 24-hour cycle, showcasing additional layers of biological complexity.

These rhythms exert influence over various bodily systems, including digestion, immunity, cognition, and cardiovascular function. For instance, fluctuations in digestive and absorptive capacities throughout the day can impact the efficiency of nutrient processing.

Recognizing and accommodating these biological rhythms may offer health benefits. Practices such as the Circadian Diet, which advocate for normal sleep patterns and timing of meals according to the body's natural clock, exemplify approaches that leverage biological rhythms to optimize health outcomes.

The intricate network of biological rhythms, with the circadian rhythm at its core, plays a pivotal role in maintaining homeostasis and promoting health. Lifestyle choices that respect and synchronize with these rhythms have the potential to enhance overall well-being, while disruptions to these cycles can have profound consequences. Ongoing scientific research continues to shed light on the complex relationship between circadian rhythms and health, offering valuable insights to inform strategies for improving physical and mental wellness.

SECTION 2: PRINCIPLES OF THE CIRCADIAN DIET

Aligning dietary patterns with the innate circadian rhythm of the body stands as a fundamental principle within the framework of the Circadian Diet, aiming to optimize metabolic function, energy equilibrium, and overall bodily health. While the overarching objectives remain consistent across Circadian Diet guidelines, specific recommendations may vary depending on individual needs and preferences.

Central to the concept of Time-Restricted Eating (TRE) within the Circadian Diet is the practice of restricting the daily intake of food, typically within a window spanning 12 to 16 hours, followed by a designated period for eating. By implementing such a regimen, the goal is to enhance metabolic efficiency and synchronize meal times with the body's natural circadian cycle.

An emphasis within the Circadian Diet is placed on consuming more substantial, calorically dense meals during the morning hours when metabolic activity tends to peak. This approach is believed to facilitate optimal energy utilization and align with the body's inherent circadian rhythms.

Moreover, the diet advocates for the strategic timing of nutrient intake, with an emphasis on carbohydrate and protein consumption in the morning and prioritizing healthy fats in the evening. This strategy aims to harmonize food intake with the body's fluctuating energy demands throughout the day.

By harmonizing dietary habits with the body's natural circadian rhythms, which are regulated by hormones like cortisol and melatonin, the Circadian Diet endeavors to optimize overall health. This recognition of the body's internal clock underscores the importance of adjusting eating patterns to coincide with fluctuations in hormone levels throughout the day.

Additionally, maintaining adequate hydration is underscored as a vital dietary recommendation throughout the Circadian Diet. Proper hydration supports numerous physiological functions and contributes to overall well-being.

In alignment with the circadian rhythm, which typically witnesses a decline in metabolic rate as evening approaches, the Circadian Diet often advises against late-night snacking to facilitate digestion and promote restful sleep.

Furthermore, the diet prioritizes the consumption of whole, nutrient-dense foods over processed or refined alternatives, aligning with both the nutritional objectives of the Circadian Diet and broader principles of healthy eating.

While the Circadian Diet does not operate in isolation from other lifestyle factors, it acknowledges the significance of maintaining regular sleep patterns in conjunction with dietary practices. Adequate high-quality sleep is deemed essential for overall health and complements the nutritional components of the circadian rhythm.

Advocates of the Circadian Diet suggest that timing physical exercise to coincide with the body's natural sleep-wake cycle may enhance metabolic health and energy expenditure. However, it's essential to recognize that individual responses to the Circadian Diet may vary, and ongoing research in circadian nutrition continues to evolve.

In light of these considerations, it is prudent to seek guidance from healthcare professionals or certified dietitians before implementing significant changes to dietary habits, as with any nutritional regimen.

Understanding the Mechanisms of the Circadian Diet

The fundamental concept of the Circadian Diet revolves around harmonizing dietary patterns with the body's intrinsic circadian rhythm, a 24-hour cycle governing various physiological processes. Central to this dietary approach is the practice of Time-Restricted Eating (TRE), wherein individuals allocate a specific timeframe for consuming meals during the day, followed by a prolonged fasting period typically lasting 12 to 16 hours. The objective of TRE is to optimize metabolic function and overall health by aligning meal timing with the body's natural clock.

Meal timing is a cornerstone of the Circadian Diet, emphasizing the consumption of substantial, energy-rich meals in the morning when metabolic activity is highest. This aligns with the body's preference for calorie burning during daylight hours. Conversely, lighter meals are recommended in the evening as the body prepares for rest and recovery during the night, necessitating less energy expenditure.

In addition to meal timing, nutritional timing plays a crucial role in the Circadian Diet. It involves purposefully ingesting specific nutrients at opportune times to cater to the body's evolving dietary requirements throughout the day. Carbohydrates and protein are advocated for morning consumption when energy expenditure peaks, while healthy fats are preferred in the evening to support relaxation and metabolic processes during sleep.

The Circadian Diet also considers hormonal fluctuations, such as those influenced by melatonin and cortisol, which impact sleep-wake cycles and alertness levels. Adjusting dietary practices to coincide with these hormonal shifts, including aligning meal times with peaks in melatonin production in the evening and cortisol levels in the morning, may contribute to improved metabolic health and sleep quality.

Furthermore, the Circadian Diet extends beyond dietary choices to encompass various lifestyle factors, including regular physical activity, adequate hydration, and consistent sleep patterns. By integrating these lifestyle elements with its nutritional principles, the Circadian Diet aims to enhance overall health by optimizing the body's natural rhythm.

While the Circadian Diet offers a structured framework for dietary management, individual responses may vary. It is essential to consider personal preferences, health conditions, and specific nutritional needs when implementing dietary changes. Seeking guidance from healthcare professionals or registered dietitians can provide personalized recommendations and ensure that dietary modifications align with individual well-being.

The relationship linking Circadian Rhythms and nutrition is tightly intertwined.

The intricate interplay between diet and circadian rhythms holds profound implications for overall health and well-being. At the core of this relationship lies the body's intrinsic circadian rhythm, governing a multitude of physiological processes on a 24-hour cycle. Nowhere is this connection more evident than in the realm of nutrition, where the timing and composition of meals exert a significant influence on the body's metabolic processes and utilization of nutrients.

Circadian rhythms exert a notable impact on metabolic functions, orchestrating daily fluctuations in energy expenditure, insulin sensitivity, and nutrient absorption. Research suggests that glucose metabolism may peak in the morning, coinciding with heightened insulin sensitivity driven by the body's natural rhythms. This insight forms the basis of the Circadian Diet, advocating for larger, energy-dense meals in the morning to align with these metabolic peaks and enhance nutrient utilization.

Furthermore, circadian rhythms modulate hormones involved in appetite regulation, such as leptin and ghrelin. Disruptions to circadian rhythms, as seen in shift work or irregular sleep patterns, may dysregulate these hormones, predisposing individuals to overeating and weight gain. Thus, maintaining a consistent meal schedule in harmony with circadian rhythms is crucial for hormone management and weight maintenance.

Nutrient timing also emerges as a pivotal aspect of the diet-circadian rhythm interface. Carbohydrates and protein may be more efficiently utilized by the body during periods of heightened energy demands, while dietary fats may play a more advantageous role in the evening when metabolic activity tends to decline. Aligning nutrient intake with these inherent fluctuations in energy utilization optimizes nutrient utilization and metabolic efficiency.

Moreover, circadian rhythms influence meal timing, impacting digestion and nutrient absorption. Consistent meal timing promotes efficient nutrient absorption and utilization by synchronizing with the body's rhythmic digestive processes. Conversely, disruptions to this rhythm, such as late-night eating, can adversely affect both sleep quality and metabolic health.

Recognizing the significance of both meal timing and composition underscores the importance of integrating circadian principles into dietary recommendations. By adhering to a meal schedule that aligns with the body's biological clock, individuals may experience improvements in metabolic health, hormone regulation, and overall dietary balance. As our understanding of these relationships evolves, integrating circadian principles into public health initiatives and individual dietary guidelines holds promise for promoting optimal health and well-being.

SECTION 3: BIOLOGICAL CLOCKS AND SYNCHRONIZATION

Embedded within every living cell is a sophisticated biological timekeeper responsible for regulating a myriad of physiological and behavioral processes. In humans, the master biological clock resides within the hypothalamic suprachiasmatic nucleus (SCN), orchestrating the intricate dance of our internal rhythms. This internal timekeeper is finely tuned to external cues, with the natural light-dark cycle playing a pivotal role in synchronizing our biological clocks with the outside world. Additionally, peripheral clocks scattered throughout various bodily tissues and organs collaborate with the master clock to ensure coherence in our biological cycles.

Entrainment, the harmonious alignment of our internal clocks with environmental cues, is paramount for optimal functioning. Light, particularly sunlight, serves as a potent synchronizer for the brain's master clock, exerting its influence on our sleep-wake cycle and other circadian rhythms. Exposure to light stimulates wakefulness and alertness, especially in the morning, while darkness signals the body to prepare for restorative sleep, particularly during the evening hours.

Numerous physiological processes, including hormone production, metabolism, and immune function, hinge on the synchronized ticking of our biological clocks. Hormones like cortisol surge in the morning, promoting alertness, while melatonin levels rise in the evening, facilitating the transition to sleep. This orchestrated synchronization ensures that different bodily systems peak and ebb at optimal times throughout the day.

However, disruptions to circadian synchronization, such as irregular sleep patterns, shift work, or excessive artificial light exposure at night, can lead to circadian misalignment. This misalignment has been implicated in a host of health issues, including sleep disturbances, metabolic disorders, and increased susceptibility to chronic diseases. To mitigate these risks, strategies such as maintaining a consistent sleep-wake cycle, basking in natural light during the day, and minimizing exposure to artificial light at night can help reestablish harmony among our biological clocks.

The interplay between biological clocks and environmental signals is integral to overall health and well-being, underscoring the importance of understanding and respecting our body's natural rhythms. As research in circadian biology advances, the significance of these internal timekeepers in shaping health recommendations and lifestyle interventions is becoming increasingly recognized. By honoring the rhythms of our biological clocks, we can optimize sleep, metabolism, and overall health, paving the way for a vibrant and balanced life.

The function of hormones within the circadian system is pivotal.

The circadian system can be likened to a grand ballet performance, where hormones take on the role of principal dancers, orchestrating a symphony of physiological processes that unfold in a rhythmic 24-hour cycle. At the break of dawn, cortisol, often referred to as the "stress hormone," emerges as the star of the show, guiding the body into wakefulness with a dramatic spike in its levels. This surge in cortisol promotes heightened energy levels, increased alertness, and the mobilization of resources to kickstart the day's activities. As the day progresses, cortisol levels gradually decline, reaching their lowest point in the late afternoon. This cyclical ebb and flow of cortisol secretion aligns perfectly with the body's natural rhythms, facilitating peak activity during the day and a gradual winding down towards evening.

Working in harmony with cortisol, the sleep hormone melatonin steps onto the stage as darkness falls, signaling to the body that bedtime is approaching. Melatonin production increases as the sun sets, reaching its peak in the early hours of the morning after a night of steady secretion. This rhythmic release of melatonin not only promotes restful sleep but also helps synchronize the body's internal clock with the natural light-dark cycle, ensuring optimal functioning.

In addition to cortisol and melatonin, hormones such as insulin and growth hormone play vital roles in regulating metabolic activities and promoting overall health. Insulin sensitivity follows a diurnal pattern, with mornings typically characterized by greater sensitivity, facilitating better blood sugar regulation. Similarly, growth hormone, crucial for growth, repair, and metabolism, exhibits a pulsatile release pattern, with heightened secretion during deep sleep, underscoring the importance of the circadian clock in metabolic health.

Disruptions to the body's natural hormone rhythms, whether due to irregular sleep schedules, shift work, or exposure to artificial light at night, can have profound implications for health. Metabolic disorders, compromised immune function, and an increased risk of chronic diseases have all been linked to such disturbances. Understanding the intricate interplay between the circadian clock and hormone rhythms underscores the importance of maintaining regular sleep-wake cycles and aligning lifestyle choices with the natural light-dark cycle.

To optimize the functioning of the circadian clock and promote overall well-being, it is advisable to expose oneself to natural light during the day and minimize exposure to artificial light at night. By adopting circadian-aligned practices, informed by our evolving understanding of circadian biology, individuals can cultivate healthier habits and enhance their quality of life.

Effects of Lifestyle and Surroundings on Circadian Patterns

Circadian rhythms encompass a complex series of 24-hour cycles governing a myriad of physiological processes within our bodies, meticulously orchestrated by environmental and lifestyle cues. Among the plethora of factors influencing circadian rhythms, the impact of light exposure stands paramount. Our circadian system exhibits a profound sensitivity to natural daylight, dictating our behavioral and physiological responses accordingly. Conversely, prolonged exposure to artificial light, particularly the blue light emitted by electronic devices, during nighttime hours can disrupt our natural circadian rhythm, impeding the production of melatonin and hindering our ability to achieve restorative sleep.

The regularity of one's sleep-wake cycles plays a pivotal role in maintaining the harmony of their circadian rhythms. Individuals grappling with irregular sleep patterns, such as shift workers or those with unpredictable bedtimes, are more susceptible to circadian misalignment. This discordance in circadian rhythm synchronization can precipitate a host of adverse health outcomes, spanning from sleep disturbances and cognitive impairment to an elevated risk of metabolic and cardiovascular disorders. Establishing consistent sleep schedules and cultivating a sleep-conducive environment thus emerges as imperative strategies in nurturing the natural cadence of our circadian rhythms.

Dietary habits also exert a profound influence on circadian rhythms, modulating energy balance and metabolic processes. Aligning meal timing with our body's natural rhythm, such as consuming larger, energy-dense meals during the peak metabolic period in the morning, as advocated by the Circadian Diet, can optimize metabolic health and nutrient utilization.

Furthermore, lifestyle factors encompassing stress management, physical activity, and social engagement intricately shape our circadian rhythms. Engaging in exercise during the morning or early afternoon can bolster sleep quality and strengthen the circadian system, whereas chronic stress disrupts hormone release patterns, exacerbating circadian dysregulation. Exposure to natural daylight and social interactions during the daytime fosters positive mood and overall well-being, reinforcing the symbiotic relationship between circadian rhythms and lifestyle variables.

In essence, the delicate equilibrium of circadian rhythms is profoundly influenced by environmental cues and lifestyle choices. Adopting strategies such as maintaining regular sleep schedules, minimizing light exposure during nighttime hours, adhering to circadian-aligned dietary patterns, and engaging in regular physical activity constitute integral components of a holistic approach to optimizing circadian health. Embracing these behaviors as habitual practices facilitates the enhancement of energy levels and overall well-being, underscoring the significance of integrating lifestyle modifications with circadian rhythm considerations in pursuit of optimal health and wellness. As our understanding of circadian biology continues to evolve, ongoing guidance for lifestyle modifications conducive to circadian-aligned living remains crucial in fostering enduring health benefits.

SECTION 4: NUTRIENT-RICH FOODS THAT PROMOTE CIRCADIAN WELLNESS

By supplying the body with the necessary vitamins, minerals, and macronutrients for optimum function at different times of the day, nutrient-dense meals significantly contribute to circadian health. The Circadian Diet is based on the idea that eating in sync with the body's natural circadian cycle will improve metabolic efficiency and general health.

A nutrient-dense meal eaten first thing in the morning can provide you energy to go through the day. Complex carbohydrate foods, such fruits, vegetables, and whole grains, can provide a consistent supply of glucose, which can aid with mental acuity and alertness. The amino acids needed for muscle repair and neurotransmitter production can be found in protein sources such as eggs, yogurt, or lean meats.

Maintaining an emphasis on nutritional density throughout the day is important for both meals and snacks. To feel full on fewer calories and keep blood sugar levels stable, eat lean meats, veggies high in fiber, and healthy fats like nuts and avocados. These nutrient-dense choices may keep you going all day long, unlike less balanced meals that tend to leave you feeling sluggish in the middle.

Later in the day, you should go for lighter, more digestible fare. Without putting too much strain on the digestive system, critical nutrients can still be provided via vegetables, lean proteins, and complex carbs. In order to promote metabolic health and be in sync with the body's natural circadian rhythm, some who follow the Circadian Diet recommend cutting back on late-night snacks.

To maintain proper circadian health, it is essential to drink enough of water and eat enough of water-rich meals, such as fruits and vegetables. Digestion, vitamin absorption, and detoxification are just a few of the physiological processes that benefit from maintaining a sufficient water intake.

The foundation of circadian health is nutrient-dense meals, but it's important to take into account personal dietary choices, limitations, and health issues. In general, it is advised to eat whole, minimally processed meals that offer a balanced combination of carbs, proteins, fats, vitamins, and minerals. A well-rounded and long-term strategy for circadian-aligned eating can be achieved by seeking the advice of a healthcare provider or certified dietitian, as is the case with any dietary plan.

The significance of maintaining adequate hydration within the Circadian Diet

Within the framework of the body's innate circadian rhythm, maintaining adequate hydration emerges as a pivotal aspect of the Circadian Diet, exerting profound effects on overall health and well-being. While the primary function of water is to hydrate the body, its significance extends far beyond mere replenishment, intricately woven into the core functions of the circadian system such as metabolism, digestion, and detoxification.

Following a night's rest, during which water is lost through respiration and perspiration, it becomes imperative to rehydrate upon awakening to offset these losses. By kickstarting the metabolism and replenishing lost fluids, consuming water in the morning can invigorate and energize the body, setting the stage for a productive day ahead. Aligning with the Circadian Diet's principles, prioritizing hydration in the morning helps sustain the body's heightened metabolic rate throughout the day.

Furthermore, maintaining optimal hydration levels throughout the day facilitates the processes of nutrient absorption and transportation, thus supporting the body's circadian rhythm. Adequate hydration is integral to the digestive system's ability to break down food and extract nutrients efficiently. Moreover, water plays a crucial role in regulating core body temperature, which undergoes cyclical changes as dictated by the circadian rhythm. By ensuring adequate hydration, individuals can aid their bodies in adapting to these temperature fluctuations and promoting optimal thermoregulation.

However, it is advisable to exercise caution when hydrating in the evening to avoid disruptions to sleep patterns. While staying hydrated remains paramount, consuming smaller quantities of fluids closer to bedtime can help minimize nocturnal awakenings due to bathroom trips, thus promoting uninterrupted sleep. This approach, endorsed by the Circadian Diet, underscores the importance of harmonizing hydration patterns with the body's natural circadian cycle to optimize sleep quality.

Moreover, the choice of hydrating beverages is integral to adhering to the principles of the Circadian Diet. While herbal teas and infusions offer variety, opting for caffeine-free options aligns with the diet's focus on enhancing sleep hygiene. Nonetheless, water remains the preferred choice for hydration, particularly in light of its alignment with the body's circadian rhythm.

Directionss for Aligning with Circadian Rhythms through Daily Habits

To optimize your well-being, it's advisable to harmonize your daily activities with your body's innate circadian rhythm, a practice known as circadian alignment. The cornerstone of this approach lies in maintaining a consistent sleep-wake schedule. By adhering to a regular bedtime and waking up time each day, you reinforce your body's internal clock, thereby enhancing the quality and duration of your sleep. This consistent sleep pattern supports circadian alignment and facilitates crucial restorative processes associated with sleep, such as hormone regulation and cellular repair.

Exposure to sunlight throughout the day plays a pivotal role in regulating sleep-wake cycles. Natural light serves as a potent signal for the circadian clock, influencing sleep patterns, mood, and alertness. Maximizing exposure to sunlight, particularly in the morning, aids in circadian entrainment, helping synchronize your body's internal clock. Conversely, it's essential to minimize nighttime exposure to artificial light, particularly blue light emitted by screens, as this can suppress melatonin production, signaling the brain that it's time to prepare for sleep.

Engaging in physical activity at strategic times can also help maintain circadian rhythms. Regular exercise, particularly in the morning or early evening, can promote better sleep quality and daytime alertness by positively influencing the circadian clock. However, vigorous exercise close to bedtime may have the opposite effect, as it can elevate cortisol levels, making it more challenging for the body to wind down for sleep.

Mindful eating practices, such as those advocated by the Circadian Diet, also contribute to circadian synchronization. This dietary approach emphasizes timing meals to coincide with the body's natural metabolic fluctuations. Consuming larger, more energy-dense meals earlier in the day and lighter meals later in the day helps reinforce the influence of the circadian rhythm on metabolism.

Stress management and relaxation techniques are integral components of a circadian-aligned lifestyle. Chronic stress can disrupt hormonal rhythms and impair sleep quality, underscoring the importance of incorporating practices like meditation, deep breathing, and gentle yoga to promote harmony between body and mind within the context of the natural daily rhythms.

Additionally, fostering social connections and adhering to a consistent daily routine further supports circadian synchronization. Human interactions and established routines provide a sense of stability and predictability, strengthening the body's internal clock and promoting overall well-being.

As our understanding of circadian biology continues to evolve, it becomes increasingly evident how lifestyle behaviors can be leveraged to align with our natural rhythms, ultimately facilitating optimal health and vitality. By integrating these principles into our daily lives, we can cultivate a harmonious relationship with our bodies and unlock the full potential of circadian-aligned living.

SECTION 5: DISTINCTIVE FACTORS AND DIVERSE MODIFICATIONS

When crafting circadian-aligned routines, it's essential to consider each individual's distinct characteristics, lifestyle preferences, and current health status. Central to this consideration is the recognition of chronotypes, or the innate predispositions individuals have toward certain times of day.

Some naturally gravitate towards being "morning people," while others resonate more with the identity of "night owls." Optimizing the effectiveness of circadian-aligned living involves tailoring practices to align with one's chronotype. For instance, individuals who feel most alert in the morning may find it beneficial to prioritize essential tasks during this time, whereas those inclined towards nocturnal energy may thrive by scheduling activities, such as exercise, in the evening.

Shift workers face additional challenges in harmonizing their daily routines with their circadian rhythms due to irregular work schedules. Establishing a consistent sleep schedule, ensuring exposure to adequate light during work hours, and practicing good sleep hygiene become imperative strategies for this population. Employers can play a supportive role by fostering healthy work environments and considering circadian principles when organizing shift patterns.

Age also plays a significant role in circadian rhythms, with adolescents experiencing a natural shift towards later sleep onset and waking times. Recognizing these age-related differences and adapting school or work schedules accordingly can contribute to the overall well-being of this demographic.

Health conditions and medications can further influence circadian rhythms, necessitating tailored interventions to address circadian misalignments associated with sleep disorders or mood disturbances. Healthcare providers play a crucial role in providing personalized guidance to individuals navigating these challenges, ensuring that circadian considerations are integrated into treatment strategies.

While the Circadian Diet and lifestyle recommendations offer broad guidelines for circadian alignment, it's essential to acknowledge the diversity of human experiences and the influence of cultural, social, and occupational factors. Flexibility in applying circadian practices allows individuals to customize these concepts to their unique circumstances.

Perspectives and insights from experts in the field.

Gaining a comprehensive understanding and effectively applying circadian-aligned Directionsologies is greatly enhanced by incorporating professional perspectives and insights from various domains. From a medical standpoint, the expertise of chronobiologists and sleep medicine specialists proves invaluable in diagnosing and treating circadian rhythm disorders. Drawing upon their extensive knowledge of how disruptions to the normal circadian cycle impact health, these professionals may recommend interventions such as light therapy, melatonin supplementation, or adjustments to sleep patterns to promote circadian alignment and overall well-being.

In the realm of dietary practices, the Circadian Diet benefits from the input of nutritionists and dietitians who emphasize the importance of meal timing and composition. Their expert recommendations on the types and timing of meals conducive to circadian health are informed by a deep understanding of nutritional science. By tailoring dietary advice to synchronize with the body's natural rhythms, these specialists play a crucial role in fostering metabolic efficiency and supporting overall health.

Occupational health specialists and workplace strategists offer a fresh perspective on circadian-aligned activities, particularly for individuals working irregular hours or shifts. Their insights inform the development of policies and practices aimed at promoting employee health and circadian well-being in the workplace. This may include designing work environments that accommodate circadian rhythms, optimizing break schedules, and implementing strategies to mitigate the negative effects of shift work on health.

Researchers in the field of circadian biology continually expand our understanding of the complex mechanisms underlying circadian rhythms. Their work investigates the impact of circadian disturbances on various aspects of health and wellness, providing crucial evidence for evidence-based treatments and lifestyle recommendations. By bridging the gap between theoretical understanding and practical implementation, these researchers play a vital role in helping individuals align their routines with their natural circadian rhythms.

Psychological insights from mental health specialists and psychologists offer valuable perspectives on the psychological components of living in sync with one's circadian rhythm. Their research explores the connections between circadian cycles and factors such as stress, mood, and overall psychological well-being. By addressing issues such as stress management, resilience, and the formation of healthy habits conducive to mental health, these professionals contribute to a more holistic approach to circadian routines.

By integrating expert opinions from various disciplines, circadian-aligned lifestyles can be more effectively designed and implemented, addressing not only physical but also mental, social, and ecological aspects of well-being. Interdisciplinary collaboration fosters the development of holistic approaches that cater to individual needs and preferences, ultimately helping individuals achieve their health and vitality goals. As circadian principles become increasingly integrated into conventional healthcare and lifestyle practices, we can expect to see a shift towards more personalized and holistic approaches to health and wellness.

SECTION 6: CIRCADIAN DIET DISHES YOU SHOULD DEFINITELY TRY

CIRCADIAN DIET BREAKFAST RECOMMENDATIONS

Healthy porridge bowl

What You Need

100g frozen raspberries

1 orange, ½ sliced and ½ juiced

150g porridge oats

100ml milk

½ banana, sliced

2 tbsp smooth almond butter

1 tbsp goji berries

1 tbsp chia seeds

Directions

STEP 1

Tip half the raspberries and all of the orange juice in a pan. Simmer until the raspberries soften, about 5 mins.

STEP 2

Meanwhile stir the oats, milk and 450ml water in a pan over a low heat until creamy. Top with the raspberry compote, remaining raspberries, orange slices, banana, almond butter, goji berries and chia seeds.

One-pan eggs & peppers

What You Need

1 tbsp olive oil

2 onions (320g), halved and thinly sliced

1 orange pepper, halved, deseeded and sliced

1 red chilli, deseeded and sliced

400g can chopped tomatoes

2 tbsp tomato purée

2 tsp vegetable bouillon powder

1 tsp dried oregano

1 tsp smoked paprika, plus a little for sprinkling

2 x 400g cans chickpeas

4 eggs

2 x 120g pots bio yogurt

2 garlic cloves, finely grated

4 tbsp chopped parsley

Directions

STEP 1

Heat the oil over a medium heat in a large deep frying pan with a lid. Stir in the onions, then cover and leave to cook for 5 mins. Remove the lid and give the onions a stir – they should have softened and be starting to brown in places. Stir in the pepper and chilli, and cook for 2 mins, then tip in the tomatoes, tomato purée, bouillon, oregano, paprika and chickpeas, along with their liquid. Cover and turn the heat down to a simmer for 15 mins.

STEP 2

Create two dips in the mixture with a spoon and crack 2 eggs into them. Cover and cook over a low heat for about 5 mins, until just set.

STEP 3

Meanwhile, stir the yogurt with the garlic in a small bowl and sprinkle with paprika. Serve half the chickpea mixture with the cooked eggs. Serve half the yogurt on the side and sprinkle with half the parsley and a little paprika. Cool and chill the remainder. Will keep covered in the fridge for five days.

Chocolate porridge

What You Need

125g porridge oats

4 dates, stoned

500-600ml milk, any will work

1 tbsp cacao or good quality cocoa powder

yogurt and maple syrup, to serve (optional)

Directions

STEP 1

Blend half the oats and the dates in a food processor until you have a thick paste, adding a splash of milk to help the blades go round if necessary. Scrape the mixture into a saucepan and add the rest of the oats, 500ml milk, the cacao and a pinch of salt. Stir well and set over a low-medium heat.

STEP 2

Stir the porridge every now and then for the next 5-10 mins, until it's thick and creamy – add a splash more milk if you prefer a looser consistency. Serve with a dollop of yogurt and a drizzle of maple syrup, if you like.

Green spirulina smoothie

What You Need

½ small avocado, peeled and stoned

1 tsp spirulina powder

50g baby spinach

¼ cucumber, roughly chopped

1 lime, zested and juiced

10g mint, plus a sprig to garnish (optional)

75ml apple juice (not from concentrate), chilled

1 tsp honey (optional)

Directions

STEP 1

Tip all the What You Need into a blender or food processor with 75ml cold water, and blitz until smooth. Or, put everything in a bowl and blitz with a hand blender.

STEP 2

Pour into a tall glass and garnish with a mint sprig, if you like. Drink straightaway

Walnut & almond muesli with grated apple

What You Need

85g porridge oats

15g flaked almonds

15g walnuts,chopped

15g pumpkin seeds

1 tsp ground cinnamon

80g raisins

15g high fibre puffed wheat (we used Good Grain)

4 apples, no need to peel, grated

fortified oat milk, to serve

Directions

STEP 1

Put the porridge oats in a saucepan and heat gently, stirring frequently until they're just starting to toast. Turn off the heat, then add all of the nuts, pumpkin seeds, and cinnamon, then stir everything together well.

STEP 2

Tip into a large bowl, stir to help it cool, then add the raisins and puffed wheat and toss together until well mixed. Tip half into a jar or airtight container and save for another day – it will keep at room temperature. Serve the rest in two bowls, grate over 2 apples and pour over some cold cold milk (you can also use regular or preferred non-dairy milk) at the table. Save the other apples for the remaining muesli.

Mushroom hash with poached eggs

What You Need

1 ½ tbsp avocado oil

2 large onions, halved and sliced

500g closed cup mushrooms, quartered

1 tbsp fresh thyme leaves, plus extra for sprinkling

500g fresh tomatoes, chopped

1 tsp smoked paprika

4 tsp omega seed mix (see tip)

4 large eggs

Directions

STEP 1

Heat the oil in a large non-stick frying pan and fry the onions for a few mins. Cover the pan and leave the onions to cook in their own steam for 5 mins more.

STEP 2

Tip in the mushrooms with the thyme and cook, stirring frequently, for 5 mins until softened. Add the tomatoes and paprika, cover the pan and cook for 5 mins until pulpy. Stir through the seed mix.

STEP 3

If you're making this recipe as part of our two-person Summer Healthy Diet Plan, poach two of the eggs in lightly simmering water to your liking. Serve on top of half the hash with a sprinkling of fresh thyme and some black pepper. Chill the remaining hash to warm in a pan and eat with freshly poached eggs on another day. If you're serving four people, poach all four eggs, divide the hash between four plates, sprinkle with thyme and black pepper and serve with the eggs on top.

Apple & linseed porridge

What You Need

100g porridge oat

2 eating apples, peeled and grated

½ tsp ground cinnamon, plus extra for sprinkling

500ml skimmed milk

2 tbsp ground linseed

150ml pot probiotic yogurt

drizzle of honey or agave syrup

Directions

STEP 1

In a medium saucepan, mix the oats, apples, cinnamon and milk. Bring to the boil, stirring occasionally, then turn down the heat and cook for 4-5 mins, stirring constantly.

STEP 2

Stir in the ground linseeds, then divide into 4 breakfast bowls. Top each with a dollop of yogurt, a drizzle of honey or agave syrup, and a sprinkle more cinnamon

Sweet potato pancakes with orange & grapefruit

What You Need

325g sweet potatoes, peeled and coarsely grated

½ tsp vanilla extract

2 oranges, 1 zested, both cut into segments

150g ricotta or bio yogurt

2 large eggs

½ tsp baking powder

2 tsp rapeseed oil

2 grapefruits, cut into segments

small handful mint leaves

Directions

STEP 1

Put the sweet potato in a bowl, cover with cling film and cook in the microwave on high for 5 mins (or steam them). Mash the potato with a fork. When cooled a little, beat in the vanilla, orange zest, ricotta, eggs and baking powder to make a batter.

STEP 2

Heat the oil in a non-stick frying pan and fry spoonfuls of the batter for a few mins. Carefully flip the pancakes to cook the other side. When done, set aside on a plate and cook the remaining batter, aiming for eight pancakes in total.

STEP 3

If you are following our Healthy Diet Plan, you should serve four on the first day and set aside four for another day – keep in the fridge and reheat in a microwave or in a pan. Alternatively, cook half the batter now, reserving the rest for another day – but you will need to add ¼ tsp baking powder to the mixture before using it.

STEP 4

Mix the grapefruit and orange segments with mint and serve with the pancakes.

Better-than-baked beans with spicy wedges

What You Need

1 tsp oil

1 onion, halved and thinly sliced

2 rashers streaky bacon, cut into large-ish pieces

1 tsp sugar, brown if you have it

400g can chopped tomato

200ml stock from a cube

410g can cannellini bean, butter or haricot beans in water

For the wedges

1 tbsp white flour (plain or self-raising)

0.5 tsp cayenne pepper, paprika or mild chilli powder

1 tsp dried mixed herb (optional)

2 baking potatoes, each cut into 8 wedges

2 tsp oil

Directions

STEP 1

Heat oven to 200C/fan 180C/gas 6. For the wedges, mix the flour, cayenne and herbs (if using), add some salt and pepper, then toss with the potatoes and oil until well coated. Tip into a roasting tin, then bake for about 35 mins until crisp and cooked through.

STEP 2

Meanwhile, heat the oil in a non-stick pan, then gently fry the onion and bacon together for 5-10 mins until the onions are softened and just starting to turn golden. Stir in the sugar, tomatoes, stock and seasoning to taste, then simmer the sauce for 5 mins. Add the beans, then simmer for another 5 mins until the sauce has thickened. Serve with the wedges.

Date & buckwheat granola with pecans & seeds

What You Need

For the granola

85g buckwheat

4 medjool dates, stoned

1 tsp ground cinnamon

100g traditional oats

2 tsp rapeseed oil

25g sunflower seeds

25g pumpkin seeds

25g flaked almonds

50g pecan nuts, roughly broken into halves

50g sultanas (without added oil)

For the yogurt & fruit (to serve 2)

2 x 150ml pots low-fat bio natural yogurt

2 ripe nectarines or peaches, stoned and sliced

Directions

STEP 1

Soak the buckwheat overnight in cold water. The next day, drain and rinse the buckwheat. Put the dates in a pan with 300ml water and the cinnamon, and blitz with a stick blender until completely smooth. Add the buckwheat, bring to the boil and cook, uncovered, for 5 mins until pulpy. Meanwhile, heat oven to 150C/130C fan/gas 2 and line two large baking trays with baking parchment.

STEP 2

Stir the oats and oil into the date and buckwheat mixture, then spoon small clusters of the mixture onto the baking trays. Bake for 15 mins, then carefully scrape the clusters from the parchment if they have stuck and turn before spreading out again. Return to the oven for another 15 mins, turning frequently, until firm and golden.

STEP 3

When the mix is dry enough, tip into a bowl, mix in the seeds and nuts with the sultanas and toss well. When cool, serve each person a generous handful with yogurt and fruit, and pack the excess into an airtight container. Will keep for a week. On other days you can vary the fruit or serve with milk or a dairy-free alternative instead of the yogurt.

Spiced oatmeal fritters with coconut caramel pears

What You Need

250ml almond milk

½ tsp ground cloves

1 tsp ground nutmeg

4 tsp ground cinnamon

100g rolled oats

3 large eggs

For the caramel pears

2 tbsp golden caster sugar

75g coconut butter

2 firm Williams pears, peeled, cored and thinly sliced

200g coconut yogurt, to serve

Directions

STEP 1

In a large saucepan, combine the almond milk, cloves, nutmeg and 3 tsp of the cinnamon. Bring to a simmer. Tip in the oats and cook for 6 mins over a low heat, stirring constantly, until thick and creamy, like porridge. Scrape into a mixing bowl, cover, and cool for 20 mins.

STEP 2

While you wait, make the caramel pears. Sprinkle the sugar evenly over a frying pan set on a low heat. Don't stir it, but wait until it starts to melt, turning dark golden here and there. When most of the sugar is melted, gently swirl to incorporate any dry patches. Stir in 25g of the coconut butter. Toss the pear slices in the remaining cinnamon, then add to the caramel and cook for 5 mins until softened. Set aside.

STEP 3

Return to the oats now, beating in the eggs and ½ tsp salt to make a loose pancake-like batter.

Heat oven to 140C/120C fan/gas 1 and put plates in to warm.

STEP 4

Melt a little of the remaining coconut butter in a frying pan. When hot, add half-ladlefuls of the batter spaced apart and cook for 4 mins each side, or until golden brown. Remove to a plate and keep warm in the oven. Continue frying the fritters, adding more coconut butter as needed. Serve the fritters topped with a spoonful of coconut yogurt followed by the warm pears.

Tofu scramble

What You Need

1 tbsp olive oil

1 small onion, finely sliced

1 large garlic clove, crushed

½ tsp turmeric

1 tsp ground cumin

½ tsp sweet smoked paprika

280g extra firm tofu

100g cherry tomatoes, halved

½ small bunch parsley, chopped

rye bread, to serve, (optional)

Directions

STEP 1

Heat the oil in a frying pan over a medium heat and gently fry the onion for 8 -10 mins or until golden brown and sticky. Stir in the garlic, turmeric, cumin and paprika and cook for 1 min.

STEP 2

Roughly mash the tofu in a bowl using a fork, keeping some pieces chunky. Add to the pan and fry for 3 mins. Raise the heat, then tip in the tomatoes, cooking for 5 mins more or until they begin to soften. Fold the parsley through the mixture. Serve on its own or with toasted rye bread (not gluten-free), if you like

Mushroom hash with poached eggs

What You Need

1 ½ tbsp avocado oil

2 large onions, halved and sliced

500g closed cup mushrooms, quartered

1 tbsp fresh thyme leaves, plus extra for sprinkling

500g fresh tomatoes, chopped

1 tsp smoked paprika

4 tsp omega seed mix (see tip)

4 large eggs

Directions

STEP 1

Heat the oil in a large non-stick frying pan and fry the onions for a few mins. Cover the pan and leave the onions to cook in their own steam for 5 mins more.

STEP 2

Tip in the mushrooms with the thyme and cook, stirring frequently, for 5 mins until softened. Add the tomatoes and paprika, cover the pan and cook for 5 mins until pulpy. Stir through the seed mix.

STEP 3

If you're making this recipe as part of our two-person Summer Healthy Diet Plan, poach two of the eggs in lightly simmering water to your liking. Serve on top of half the hash with a sprinkling of fresh thyme and some black pepper. Chill the remaining hash to warm in a pan and eat with freshly poached eggs on another day. If you're serving four people, poach all four eggs, divide the hash between four plates, sprinkle with thyme and black pepper and serve with the eggs on top.

Socca pancakes with hummus & lemony onions

What You Need

75g gram (chickpea) flour

2 tsp rapeseed or olive oil

For the topping

1 red onion, halved and thinly sliced

½ lemon, juiced

4 tbsp hummus

2 tomatoes, cut into wedges

3 small coriander sprigs

2 handfuls mixed salad leaves

Directions

STEP 1

Mix the flour with 180ml water until fully combined. If you have time, leave to stand for 30 mins. Meanwhile, toss the onion with the lemon juice in a separate bowl.

STEP 2

Heat 1 tsp of the oil in a large non-stick frying pan over a low heat and pour in half the batter. Swirl the pan to coat the base evenly and cook for about 6 mins until firm and you can lift the edge of the pancake off the pan. Using a spatula or palette knife, turn the pancake over and cook for 4-6 mins on the other side, until cooked through and crisp at the edge. Keep warm in a low oven while you cook the second pancake in the same way.

STEP 3

Spread hummus down the middle of each pancake, then top with the tomatoes, quick-pickled onions, coriander and salad leaves. Fold in half to serve

Sweet potato pancakes with orange & grapefruit

What You Need

325g sweet potatoes, peeled and coarsely grated

½ tsp vanilla extract

2 oranges, 1 zested, both cut into segments

150g ricotta or bio yogurt

2 large eggs

½ tsp baking powder

2 tsp rapeseed oil

2 grapefruits, cut into segments

small handful mint leaves

Directions

STEP 1

Put the sweet potato in a bowl, cover with cling film and cook in the microwave on high for 5 mins (or steam them). Mash the potato with a fork. When cooled a little, beat in the vanilla, orange zest, ricotta, eggs and baking powder to make a batter.

STEP 2

Heat the oil in a non-stick frying pan and fry spoonfuls of the batter for a few mins. Carefully flip the pancakes to cook the other side. When done, set aside on a plate and cook the remaining batter, aiming for eight pancakes in total.

STEP 3

If you are following our Healthy Diet Plan, you should serve four on the first day and set aside four for another day – keep in the fridge and reheat in a microwave or in a pan. Alternatively, cook half the batter now, reserving the rest for another day – but you will need to add ¼ tsp baking powder to the mixture before using it.

STEP 4

Mix the grapefruit and orange segments with mint and serve with the pancakes.

Date & buckwheat granola with pecans & seeds

What You Need

For the granola

85g buckwheat

4 medjool dates, stoned

1 tsp ground cinnamon

100g traditional oats

2 tsp rapeseed oil

25g sunflower seeds

25g pumpkin seeds

25g flaked almonds

50g pecan nuts, roughly broken into halves

50g sultanas (without added oil)

For the yogurt & fruit (to serve 2)

2 x 150ml pots low-fat bio natural yogurt

2 ripe nectarines or peaches, stoned and sliced

Directions

STEP 1

Soak the buckwheat overnight in cold water. The next day, drain and rinse the buckwheat. Put the dates in a pan with 300ml water and the cinnamon, and blitz with a stick blender until completely smooth. Add the buckwheat, bring to the boil and cook, uncovered, for 5 mins until pulpy. Meanwhile, heat oven to 150C/130C fan/gas 2 and line two large baking trays with baking parchment.

STEP 2

Stir the oats and oil into the date and buckwheat mixture, then spoon small clusters of the mixture onto the baking trays. Bake for 15 mins, then carefully scrape the clusters from the parchment if they have stuck and turn before spreading out again. Return to the oven for another 15 mins, turning frequently, until firm and golden.

STEP 3

When the mix is dry enough, tip into a bowl, mix in the seeds and nuts with the sultanas and toss well. When cool, serve each person a generous handful with yogurt and fruit, and pack the excess into an airtight container. Will keep for a week. On other days you can vary the fruit or serve with milk or a dairy-free alternative instead of the yogurt

Spiced oatmeal fritters with coconut caramel pears

What You Need

250ml almond milk

½ tsp ground cloves

1 tsp ground nutmeg

4 tsp ground cinnamon

100g rolled oats

3 large eggs

For the caramel pears

2 tbsp golden caster sugar

75g coconut butter

2 firm Williams pears, peeled, cored and thinly sliced

200g coconut yogurt, to serve

Directions

STEP 1

In a large saucepan, combine the almond milk, cloves, nutmeg and 3 tsp of the cinnamon. Bring to a simmer. Tip in the oats and cook for 6 mins over a low heat, stirring constantly, until thick and creamy, like porridge. Scrape into a mixing bowl, cover, and cool for 20 mins.

STEP 2

While you wait, make the caramel pears. Sprinkle the sugar evenly over a frying pan set on a low heat. Don't stir it, but wait until it starts to melt, turning dark golden here and there. When most of the sugar is melted, gently swirl to incorporate any dry patches. Stir in 25g of the coconut butter. Toss the pear slices in the remaining cinnamon, then add to the caramel and cook for 5 mins until softened. Set aside.

STEP 3

Return to the oats now, beating in the eggs and ½ tsp salt to make a loose pancake-like batter. Heat oven to 140C/120C fan/gas 1 and put plates in to warm.

STEP 4

Melt a little of the remaining coconut butter in a frying pan. When hot, add half-ladlefuls of the batter spaced apart and cook for 4 mins each side, or until golden brown. Remove to a plate and keep warm in the oven. Continue frying the fritters, adding more coconut butter as needed. Serve the fritters topped with a spoonful of coconut yogurt followed by the warm pears.

CIRCADIAN DIET LUNCH RECOMMENDATIONS

Steamed trout with mint & dill dressing

What You Need

120g new potatoes, halved

170g pack asparagus spears, woody ends trimmed

1 ½ tsp vegetable bouillon powder made up to 225ml with water

80g fine green beans, trimmed

80g frozen peas

2 skinless trout fillets

2 slices lemon

For the dressing

4 tbsp bio yogurt

1 tsp cider vinegar

¼ tsp English mustard powder

1 tsp finely chopped mint

2 tsp chopped dill

Directions

STEP 1

Put the new potatoes on to simmer in a pan of boiling water until tender. Cut the asparagus in half to shorten the spears and slice the ends without the tips. Tip the bouillon into a wide non-stick pan. Add the asparagus and beans, then cover and cook for 5 mins.

STEP 2

Add the peas to the pan, then top with the trout and lemon slices. Cover again and cook for 5 mins more until the fish flakes really easily, but is still juicy.

STEP 3

Meanwhile, mix the yogurt with the vinegar, mustard powder, mint and dill. Stir in 2-3 tbsp of the fish cooking juices. Put the veg and any remaining pan juices in bowls, top with the fish and herb dressing, then serve with the potatoes

Roasted asparagus & pea salad

What You Need

3 tbsp natural yogurt

1 tsp wholegrain mustard

½ tsp honey

½ lemon, zested and juiced

100g watercress

1 large slice sourdough bread

200g asparagus, tough ends removed

1 ½ tbsp cold-pressed rapeseed oil

2 eggs

200g frozen peas

Directions

STEP 1

Heat oven to 220C/200C fan/gas 7. Mix the yogurt, mustard and honey together. Add the lemon zest, then add the juice and some seasoning to taste. Squeeze any remaining lemon juice over the watercress.

STEP 2

Tear the bread into rough chunks and put them on a large roasting tray with the asparagus. Toss both in the rapeseed oil and seasoning, and roast for 10 mins until the asparagus is tender and croutons are golden.

STEP 3

Meanwhile, cook the eggs in a pan of boiling water for 6 mins, then add the frozen peas and cook for 1 min more. Drain and rinse both under cold water until cool. Peel the eggs, then cut into quarters.

STEP 4

To assemble, mix the asparagus and peas through the watercress, then toss through the creamy dressing. Nestle in the eggs and croutons, and serve.

Bombay potato frittata

What You Need

4 new potatoes, sliced into 5mm rounds

100g baby spinach, chopped

1 tbsp rapeseed oil

1 onion, halved and sliced

1 large garlic clove, finely grated

½ tsp ground coriander

½ tsp ground cumin

¼ tsp black mustard seeds

¼ tsp turmeric

3 tomatoes, roughly chopped

2 large eggs

½ green chilli, deseeded and finely chopped

1 small bunch of coriander, finely chopped

1 tbsp mango chutney

3 tbsp fat-free Greek yogurt

Directions

STEP 1

Cook the potatoes in a pan of boiling water for 6 mins, or until tender. Drain and leave to steam-dry. Meanwhile, put the spinach in a heatproof bowl with 1 tbsp water. Cover and microwave for 3 mins on high, or until wilted.

STEP 2

Heat the rapeseed oil in a medium non-stick frying pan. Add the onion and cook over a medium heat for 10 mins until golden and sticky. Stir in the garlic, ground coriander, ground cumin, mustard seeds and turmeric, and cook for 1 min more. Add the tomatoes and wilted spinach and cook for another 3 mins, then add the potatoes.

STEP 3

Heat the grill to medium. Lightly beat the eggs with the chilli and most of the fresh coriander and pour over the potato mixture. Grill for 4-5 mins, or until golden and just set, with a very slight wobble in the middle.

STEP 4

Leave to cool, then slice into wedges. Mix the mango chutney, yogurt and remaining fresh coriander together. Serve with the frittata wedges.

Spinach falafel & hummus bowl

What You Need

150g baby spinach

½ cucumber, sliced

1 red onion, finely sliced

4 wholemeal pittas, toasted, to serve

For the falafel

150g baby spinach

400g can chickpeas, drained

1 garlic clove, chopped

1 tsp ground cumin

½ small bunch of parsley, finely chopped

2 tbsp plain flour

1 tbsp olive oil, plus extra for rolling

For the hummus

400g chickpeas, drained

40ml olive oil, plus extra to serve

1 garlic clove, roughly chopped

1 lemon, juiced, plus extra to serve (optional)

2 tbsp tahini

Directions

STEP 1

Heat the oven to 190C/170C fan/gas 5. Line a baking sheet with non-stick parchment. Put all the falafel What You Need, except for the oil, in a food processor and season lightly. Pulse until you have a rough mix.

STEP 2

Oil your hands lightly, then take tablespoons of the falafel mix, roll into around 16 balls and put on the baking sheet. Press each one down slightly with the palm of your hand. Brush using the 1 tbsp oil and bake for 20-25 mins until firm and golden, turning halfway through.

STEP 3

While the falafel is cooking, make the hummus. Put all of the hummus What You Need into a food processor with 50ml of water and blitz until smooth and silky.

STEP 4

Put the spinach, cucumber, red onion and falafel in different sections of each bowl, alongside some hummus, then drizzle with the extra olive oil. Grind over some black pepper. Serve with the pittas on the side and more lemon for squeezing over, if you like

Cumin roast veg with tahini dressing

What You Need

3 large carrots, roughly chopped

3 peeled raw beetroots, roughly chopped

1 sweet potato, sliced

3 red onions, cut into wedges

250g cauliflower florets

1 tsp cumin seeds

2 tbsp rapeseed oil

1 tbsp balsamic vinegar

2-3 tbsp chopped mint

2-3 tbsp chopped coriander

400g can chickpeas

2 hard-boiled eggs, halved

100g young spinach leaves

For the dressing

3 tbsp tahini

1 tbsp crunchy peanut butter

1 lemon, zested and juiced

1 tsp ground coriander

1 garlic clove, finely grated

Directions

STEP 1

Heat oven to 200C/180C fan/gas 6. Tip all of the vegetables into a large roasting tin. Add the cumin seeds, oil and balsamic vinegar, then toss together. Roast for 45-50 mins until the veg is tender and starting to char.

STEP 2

Meanwhile, mix the tahini and peanut butter with the lemon juice, coriander, garlic and about 4-5 tbsp water to make a dressing.

STEP 3

When the veg is ready, leave to cool a little. Add the mint, coriander, lemon zest and chickpeas, then toss well.

STEP 4

If you're following our Healthy Diet Plan, serve two portions now with the eggs, some dressing and half the spinach, then serve the remainder on another day without the eggs

Miso roast salmon, lentil & pomegranate salad

What You Need

80g dried puy lentils

1 tsp miso paste

2 tsp finely grated ginger

1 garlic clove, finely grated

1 lime, zested and juiced

1 tsp olive oil

½ tsp black/white sesame seeds

2 x 150g skinless wild salmon fillets

1 tsp apple cider vinegar

2 carrots, cut into fine strips with a julienne peeler or knife

60g pomegranate seeds

3 spring onions, finely sliced

handful fresh coriander, chopped

Directions

STEP 1

Heat oven to 200C/180C fan/gas 6. Cook the lentils in a pan of boiling water for 20 mins until tender. Meanwhile, mix the miso paste with 1 tsp of the ginger, the garlic, half the lime juice, the oil and sesame seeds. Put the salmon fillets on a foil-lined baking tray and spread 1 tbsp of the miso mixture over them. Roast for 10-12 mins until cooked through.

STEP 2

Tip the rest of the miso mixture into a bowl with the remaining ginger and lime juice. Add the lime zest, vinegar, carrots, pomegranate, onions and coriander. Drain the lentils and toss into the salad. Divide between two plates and add the salmon

Bean & feta spread with Greek salad salsa & oatcakes

What You Need

400g can butter beans, drained

1 lemon, ½ juiced, ½ cut into 4 wedges

2 tbsp ricotta or bio yogurt

85g feta, crumbled

1 garlic clove

12 oatcakes

For the salsa

4 tomatoes, chopped

1 medium cucumber, finely diced

1 small red onion, finely chopped

12 pitted Kalamata olives, chopped

a few chopped mint leaves (optional)

Directions

STEP 1

Tip the beans, lemon juice, ricotta, 50g feta and the garlic into a bowl and blitz with a hand blender or in a food processor to make a paste. Stir in the remaining feta and spoon the mixture into four small pots.

STEP 2

To make the salsa, stir all the What You Need together with the mint (if using) and divide into four more pots, topping with a lemon wedge. These will keep, chilled in an airtight container, for two-three days. To eat, spread the oatcakes with the bean mixture, squeeze the lemon wedges over the salads and pile generously onto the oatcakes

Herby broccoli & pea soup

What You Need

1 tbsp rapeseed oil

1 onion, finely chopped

1 large garlic clove, crushed

400g broccoli, chopped into small florets

300g frozen peas

200g chard, chopped

1l low-salt veg stock

½ small bunch of basil, chopped

small bunch of dill, chopped

1 lemon, zested and juiced

2 tbsp pumpkin seeds, toasted

Directions

STEP 1

Heat the oil in a large saucepan. Add the onion and fry for 8 mins until soft and translucent. Add the garlic and cook for 1 min more. Tip in the broccoli, peas and chard, then pour over the stock and bring the mixture to the boil. Reduce the heat to a simmer, cover and cook for 25 mins.

STEP 2

Stir through the herbs, lemon zest and juice, then blitz the soup with a stick blender until completely smooth. Ladle into bowls and serve with the toasted pumpkin seeds scattered over the top

Vegan roast spiced squash salad with tahini dressing

What You Need

320g diced butternut squash

3 red onions (320g), cut into wedges

2 tbsp rapeseed oil

2 tsp smoked paprika

1 tsp cumin seeds

2 tbsp chopped thyme

125g quinoa

½ x 85g bag kale

2 tbsp pumpkin seeds

2 tbsp tahini

2 tbsp apple cider vinegar

1 garlic clove, finely grated

2 x 400g cans lentils or borlotti beans, very well drained

50g pomegranate seeds

4 generous handfuls of rocket

Directions

STEP 1

Heat the oven to 200C/180C fan/gas 6. Tip the squash and onions onto a large baking sheet and toss with 1 tsp of the oil. Spread out and sprinkle with the paprika, cumin and thyme, then roast for 30 mins.

STEP 2

Meanwhile, cook the quinoa following pack instructions, then drain well (or the base of the salad will be too wet).

STEP 3

Add the kale to the tray of veg, sprinkle over the seeds and return to the oven for 10 mins.

STEP 4

For the dressing, mix the tahini and remaining oil with the vinegar, garlic and 2 tbsp water.

STEP 5

Put the quinoa in a bowl and toss with the lentils or beans. Pile half into a salad bowl and the rest into two lunchboxes or bowls, if you're following the Healthy Diet Plan. Divide the veg on top, then drizzle with the dressing, scatter over the pomegranate seeds and top with the rocket. Chill the other two portions for the next day. Will keep chilled for up to three days.

Minty griddled chicken & peach salad

What You Need

1 lime, zested and juiced

1 tbsp rapeseed oil

2 tbsp mint, finely chopped, plus a few leaves
to serve

1 garlic clove, finely grated

2 skinless chicken breast fillets (300g)

160g fine beans, trimmed and halved

2 peaches (200g), each cut into 8 thick wedges

1 red onion, cut into wedges

1 large Little Gem lettuce (165g), roughly shredded

½ x 60g pack rocket

1 small avocado, stoned and sliced

240g cooked new potatoes

Directions

STEP 1

Mix the lime zest and juice, oil and mint, then put half in a bowl with the garlic. Thickly slice the chicken at a slight angle, add to the garlic mixture and toss together with plenty of black pepper.

STEP 2

Cook the beans in a pan of water for 3-4 mins until just tender. Meanwhile, griddle the chicken and onion for a few mins each side until cooked and tender. Transfer to a plate, then quickly griddle the peaches. If you don't have a griddle pan, use a non-stick frying pan with a drop of oil.

STEP 3

Toss the warm beans and onion in the remaining mint mixture, and pile onto a platter or into individual shallow bowls with the lettuce and rocket. Top with the avocado, peaches and chicken and scatter over the mint. Serve with the potatoes while still warm.

Mexican salmon salad

What You Need

2 tortillas

2 tbsp olive oil

½ tsp ground coriander

3 tbsp Greek yogurt

1 tsp smoked paprika

2 salmon fillets

1 lime, zested and juiced

2 Little Gem lettuces, separated into leaves

198g can sweetcorn, drained

½small pack coriander, roughly chopped

300g pack cherry tomatoes, halved

Directions

STEP 1

Heat oven to 200C/fan 180C/gas 6. Cut the tortillas into triangles using scissors, toss in 1 tbsp of the oil and the ground coriander, season, then tip onto a lined baking sheet. Bake for 8-10 mins, turning halfway, until crisp. Set aside to cool. Heat the grill to high.

STEP 2

Mix the yogurt with the smoked paprika and some seasoning, then spoon the yogurt mixture over the salmon. Place fillets on the same baking sheet, lined with parchment, and put under the grill for 8-10 mins until the fish is blackening in places, and flakes into big chunks.

STEP 3

While the salmon is cooking, whisk the remaining olive oil with the lime zest and juice to make a dressing, season, then toss the remaining salad What You Need in the dressing. Tip onto a plate, top with the salmon chunks and tortilla chips and serve

Spaghetti puttanesca with red beans & spinach

What You Need

100g wholemeal spaghetti

1 large onion, finely chopped

1 tbsp rapeseed oil

1 red chilli, deseeded and sliced

2 garlic cloves, chopped

200g cherry tomatoes, halved

2 tsp cider vinegar

1 tbsp capers

5 Kalamata olives, halved

1 tsp smoked paprika

210g can kidney beans, drained

160g spinach leaves

small handful of chopped parsley

small handful of basil leaves

Directions

STEP 1

Cook the spaghetti in simmering water for 10-12 mins until al dente. Meanwhile, fry the onion in the oil in a large non-stick frying pan with a lid until tender and turning golden. Stir in the chilli, garlic and cherry tomatoes.

STEP 2

Add the vinegar, capers, olives and paprika with a ladleful of pasta water. Stir in the beans and cook until warmed through.

STEP 3

Add the spinach to the pasta water to wilt, then drain well. Toss with the tomato and bean mixture and the parsley and basil, then pile onto plates or in shallow bowls to serve

Curried spinach & lentil soup

What You Need

2 tbsp rapeseed oil

1 onion, finely chopped

2 large garlic cloves, crushed

¼ tsp hot chilli powder

1 tsp cumin seeds

1 tbsp medium curry powder

160g dried brown lentils

1.2l low-salt veg stock

large bunch coriander

30g unsalted cashew nuts, toasted

2 lemons, zested and juiced

500g spinach

Directions

STEP 1

Heat 1 tbsp oil in a large saucepan. Add the onion and fry for 8 mins until soft and translucent. Stir in half the garlic, the chilli, cumin and curry powder and cook for 1 min more. Add the lentils and stock, then cover and simmer for 30 mins over a medium-low heat.

STEP 2

Put the coriander, remaining oil and garlic, the cashews and lemon zest in a food processor and blitz with 1-2 tbsp water until semi-smooth. Spoon the chutney into a bowl and set aside.

STEP 3

Stir the spinach into the soup and cook for 5 mins, or until wilted. Tip half the soup into a blender and blitz until smooth, then return this to the pan. Stir through lemon juice to taste.

STEP 4

Ladle the soup into bowls and top with generous dollops of the cashew chutney

Quinoa tabbouleh

What You Need

100g dried quinoa

75g parsley, roughly chopped

300g tomatoes, cut into 1cm dice (no need to remove the seeds)

100g cucumber, cut into small dice

For the dressing

1 tbsp olive oil

2 tbsp balsamic vinegar

juice and zest 0.5 lemon

drop of vanilla extract

1 tsp rice syrup or agave

pinch of Himalayan pink salt

½ garlic clove, crushed

50g salad leaves, to serve

Directions

STEP 1

Cook the quinoa following pack instructions, then set aside to cool.

STEP 2

Make the dressing by adding the olive oil, vinegar, lemon juice, vanilla extract, rice syrup, pinch of salt and garlic into a jug and whisk until smooth. Mix this into the quinoa and mix

together with all the other What You Need.
Serve on a bed of salad leaves

Danish-style yellow split pea soup

What You Need

500g dried yellow split peas, soaked for at least
2 hrs, rinsed

2 onions, finely chopped

1 large leek, finely chopped

2 medium carrots, cut into 1cm chunks

1 small celeriac, peeled and cut into 1cm chunks

2 medium parsnips, peeled and cut into 1cm
chunks

2 litres fresh vegetable stock

2 tbsp sweet white miso

1 tsp caraway seeds

1 tsp white pepper, plus extra to serve

large pinch of ground cloves

6 thyme or oregano sprigs, tied

handful of fresh dill, chopped, to serve

rye bread, mustard and pickle, to serve (optional)

Directions

STEP 1

Drain the peas and bring to the boil in a pan of salted water. Cook for 10 mins, drain, rinse and put in a slow cooker with the remaining What You Need except the dill. Cover and cook on low for 6-8 hrs, or until everything has softened. Remove and discard the thyme.

STEP 2

Stir, adjusting the soup with 250-300ml boiled water as needed. Season to taste. Sprinkle over the dill and serve with rye bread, mustard and pickle, if you like.

Lemon & marjoram sardines with walnut & pepper dressing

What You Need

6 walnut halves

juce and zest 1 lemon

2 garlic cloves

6 butterflied sardines (see step-by-step), thawed if frozen

2 tsp marjoram or oregano, plus a few extra leaves for sprinkling

100g roasted red peppers from a jar (not in oil), drained

small drizzle of rapeseed oil

baby spinach leaves

seeds from 0.5 pomegranate

Directions

STEP 1

You can use the walnuts as they are or activate them – this makes them easier to digest. If you're activating them, pour cold water over the walnuts, add a squeeze of lemon, then leave to soak overnight at room temperature. Drain and rinse.

STEP 2

Finely grate the garlic and set aside for 10 mins to allow the enzymes to activate. Open up the sardines and smear the flesh with half the garlic. Grate over the lemon zest (reserving a little to serve) and season with black pepper. Scatter over half the marjoram or oregano, then close the sardines again.

STEP 3

Put the walnuts, remaining herbs and the peppers in a bowl. Season, then blitz to a rough purée with a blender. Add the remaining garlic and a generous squeeze of lemon from one half, and blitz again.

STEP 4

Heat a drop of oil in a large non-stick frying pan and quickly wilt the spinach, then set aside. Wipe out the pan, then heat a little more oil and cook the sardines for 2 mins each side. Arrange the spinach on two plates and top with the sardines, scatter over the pomegranate seeds, then top with the dressing. Sprinkle over the reserved lemon zest and a few herb leaves, then serve with the remaining half of the lemon, cut into wedges.

Turkish pilaf with saffron & goji berries

What You Need

2 large garlic cloves

generous pinch of saffron

3 tsp rapeseed oil

200g diced skinless turkey thigh

85g wholegrain basmati rice

½ tsp ground cinnamon

1 tsp vegetable bouillon

3 celery sticks, finely chopped

1 tbsp fresh thyme leaves

1 tbsp dried goji berries

1 medium onion, halved and very thinly sliced

100g baby spinach leaves

25g flaked almonds

Directions

STEP 1

Finely chop the garlic and set aside to activate (see tip). Meanwhile, pour 2 tbsp boiling water over the saffron and set aside to infuse. Heat 2 tsp of the oil in a large, non-stick sauté pan with a lid, then add the turkey and fry for 5 mins, stirring frequently, until it starts to brown.

STEP 2

Stir the rice and cinnamon into the pan, then pour in 400ml boiling water and the bouillon, and stir well. Add the celery, thyme, goji berries and lots of ground black pepper. Cover the pan tightly to prevent steam escaping, and cook over a low heat for 20 mins.

STEP 3

Meanwhile, heat the remaining oil in a non-stick pan and add the onion. When it starts to soften, cover the pan for 5 mins to steam it a little more. Take off the lid and slowly fry for 12-15 mins until golden, stirring frequently.

STEP 4

After the rice has cooked for 20 mins, check the water level – if the rice is still too nutty and the liquid has all been absorbed, add up to 100ml more water. Stir in the saffron, cover again, and cook for 5-10 mins until the rice is tender.

STEP 5

Add the garlic and spinach, cook briefly to wilt the leaves, then turn off the heat. Toss through the fried onions and almonds. Cover the pan and leave to rest for 5 mins before serving

Salmon, sweet potato & coriander fishcakes with tahini dressing

What You Need

1 large sweet potato

2tbsp tahini

1 lemon, 1/2 zested and juiced, 1/2 cut into wedges

coriander (stalks and all)

coriander seeds

2 skinless and boneless salmon fillets, cut into chunks

150g plain flour

2tbsp olive oil

salad, to serve

Directions

STEP 1

Peel the sweet potato and cut into rough chunks, then put in a microwaveable bowl with a splash of water. Cover with cling film, then cook on high for 8 mins. Alternatively, you can cook these on a hob for 10 minutes. Meanwhile, whisk the tahini with the lemon juice and enough water to make a thick dressing. Season and set aside.

STEP 2

Carefully remove the cling film from the sweet potato, then blitz in a food processor until mashed but not pureed. Leave to cool for 5 mins, then add the coriander and coriander seeds. Blitz to a herby mash, (be careful not to over blitz as you still want some texture) and transfer to a mixing bowl. Then add the salmon, lemon zest, flour and some seasoning. Pulse again – you want the salmon to be roughly mixed in, rather than obliterated to mush.

STEP 3

In a small bowl add the remaing flour and shape into four fishcakes, dipping into the flour to fully coat. Pop on a plate and press them down lightly to create patties. Chill in the fridge for 30 minutes. Add the remaining tbsp of olive to a large non-stick frying pan over a medium heat. Add the fishcakes and fry for 5 mins on each side until crisp and golden. Serve with the lemon wedges, tahini dressing and salad.

CIRCADIAN DIET DINNER RECOMMENDATIONS

Sausage & winter greens cannelloni

What You Need

1 tbsp olive oil

2 red onions, halved and sliced

6 pork sausages

3 garlic cloves, crushed

small bunch of thyme, leaves picked

pinch of chilli flakes

1 tbsp tomato purée

400g can plum tomatoes

200g cavolo nero or other winter greens

75g butter

75g plain flour

850ml milk

nutmeg, for grating

50g parmesan, grated

12 lasagne sheets

green salad, to serve

Directions

STEP 1

Heat the oil in a large flameproof casserole over a medium heat and cook the onions for 8-10 mins until softened and starting to caramelise. Meanwhile, squeeze the sausagemeat from the skins.

STEP 2

Push the onions to one side of the casserole, then add the sausagemeat to the other. Squash it into smaller pieces using a wooden spoon, stirring occasionally for 10-12 mins until cooked and starting to brown in places. Mix the onions back in, then add the garlic, thyme, chilli flakes and tomato purée. Cook for another 1-2 mins. Tip in the plum tomatoes, crushing them with the back of the spoon. Season and bubble for 15-20 mins until the tomatoes have broken down and the sauce has reduced to a thick ragu.

STEP 3

Put the kettle on to boil. If using cavolo nero, remove and discard the tough stalks and roughly chop the leaves. For softer veg like spinach or chard, you can leave the stalks on. Put in a colander set over the sink and pour over a kettle of just-boiled water, then rinse the leaves under cold running water until cool enough to handle. Squeeze out as much water as you can, transfer to a board and finely chop. Stir the greens into the sausage ragu, cook for 1-2 mins until any excess liquid has evaporated (the mixture should be quite dry), remove from the heat and leave to cool a little.

STEP 4

Melt the butter in a separate saucepan over a medium heat. When sizzling, stir in the flour to make a sandy paste. Whisk in

the milk, a splash at a time, until completely incorporated. When the sauce is smooth and the consistency of custard, season well, grate in a good amount of nutmeg and stir in half the parmesan. Remove from the heat and set aside.

STEP 5

Drop the lasagne sheets into a large pan of boiling salted water one at a time to prevent them sticking together, then cook for 5-6 mins, stirring until soft enough to roll up but not fully cooked through. Drain and plunge into a bowl of cold water to stop the cooking process.

STEP 6

If the béchamel sauce has thickened as it's cooled down, stir in a splash more milk. Spoon a third of the sauce over the base of a baking dish roughly 25 x 35cm. Lift a sheet of lasagne out of the bowl of cold water and lay on a board with one of the short ends facing you. Spoon a generous tbsp of the sausage ragu over one end, then roll it up to enclose the filling, making a short cannelloni – there will be a little overlapping pasta. Place it in the baking dish, then continue with the remaining ragu and lasagne sheets, arranging them in the baking dish in two rows of six cannelloni. Spoon any remaining ragu over the top, then pour over the béchamel sauce to cover all the cannelloni rolls. Sprinkle with the remaining parmesan. Will keep covered and chilled for up to two days or frozen for up to two months. Leave to cool completely first. Defrost thoroughly in the fridge overnight before cooking. Heat the oven to 200C/180C fan/gas 6, then bake the cannelloni for 40 mins until bubbling at the edges and golden brown on top. Grind over some black pepper, if you like, and serve with a crisp green salad.

Coriander roast chicken thighs with puy lentil salad

What You Need

185g puy lentils

20g ginger, peeled

30g coriander, plus extra leaves to serve

1 tsp each garam masala and ground coriander

½ tsp ground cumin

2 large whole garlic cloves, plus 1 small clove, finely grated

2 tbsp lemon juice

150g pot plain bio yogurt

6 bone-in, skinless chicken thighs

1 tbsp fresh turmeric, finely grated

1 tbsp rapeseed or olive oil, plus 1 tsp

3 red onions (325g), thickly sliced

1 large red pepper and 1 large yellow pepper, deseeded and cut into chunks

400g cauliflower, cut into small florets

1 tsp cumin seeds

Directions

STEP 1

Heat the oven to 220C/200C fan/ gas 7. Boil the lentils for 35-40 mins over a medium heat until tender.

STEP 2

Meanwhile, put the ginger, fresh coriander, garam masala, the ground coriander, ground cumin and the 2 whole garlic cloves in a large bowl with half the lemon juice and 3 tbsp of the yogurt. Blitz using a hand blender until smooth. Use 4 tbsp of the mixture to coat the chicken thighs in a large bowl. Arrange the chicken on a baking tray in a single layer.

STEP 3

Add the remaining yogurt to the remaining spice and herb mixture, along with the turmeric, 1 tsp oil, the grated garlic, 1 tbsp water and remaining lemon juice to taste. Set aside.

STEP 4

Tip the onions, peppers and cauliflower into the bowl used for the chicken, and toss with 1 tbsp oil to coat in some of the spice mix. Spread the veg out on a baking tray, then put in the oven with the chicken for 30-35 mins until the chicken is cooked through.

STEP 5

Remove the chicken and wrap in foil to keep it warm. Scatter the cumin seeds over the veg and return to the oven for 5 mins until golden.

STEP 6

To serve, drain the lentils and put in a serving bowl with the roasted veg and the remaining turmeric yogurt. Gently toss together. Serve with the chicken (taking the meat off the bones), and scatter with the extra coriander. If you're following the Healthy Diet Plan, eat half and pack up the rest to eat cold another day. Will keep chilled for up to three days or frozen for up to a month.

Quinoa chilli with avocado & coriander

What You Need

1 tbsp rapeseed oil

1 onion, sliced

2 garlic cloves, chopped

1 green pepper, chopped

½-1 tsp smoked paprika

½-1 tsp chilli powder

2 tsp cumin

2 tsp coriander

400g can chopped tomatoes

½ tsp dried oregano

2 tsp vegetable bouillon powder (check the label if you're vegan)

80g quinoa, rinsed under cold water

400g can black beans, drained and rinsed

generous handful of coriander, chopped

2 tbsp bio yogurt or coconut yogurt (optional)

1 small avocado, stoned, peeled and sliced

Directions

STEP 1

Heat the oil in a non-stick frying pan and fry the onion and garlic for 8 mins. Add the pepper and spices to taste and fry for 1 min more.

STEP 2

Tip in the tomatoes and a can of water, stir in the
oregano, bouillon and quinoa, bring to the boil, then
cover and simmer for 20 mins.

STEP 3

Stir in the black beans and cook, uncovered, for 5 mins
more. Add most of the coriander, then serve topped
with the yogurt (if using), the remaining coriander and
the avocado slices.

Curried spinach, eggs & chickpeas

What You Need

1 tbsp rapeseed oil

1 onion, thinly sliced

1 garlic clove, crushed

3cm piece ginger, peeled and grated

1 tsp ground turmeric

1 tsp ground coriander

1 tsp garam masala

1 tbsp ground cumin

450g tomatoes, chopped

400g can chickpeas, drained

1 tsp sugar

200g spinach

2 large eggs

3 tbsp natural yogurt

1 red chilli, finely sliced

½ small bunch of coriander, torn

Directions

STEP 1

Heat the oil in a large frying pan or flameproof casserole pot over a medium heat, and fry the onion for 10 mins until golden and sticky. Add the garlic, ginger, turmeric, ground coriander, garam masala, cumin and tomatoes, and fry for 2 mins more. Add the chickpeas, 100ml water and the sugar and bring to a simmer. Stir in the spinach, then cover and cook for 20-25 mins. Season to taste.

STEP 2

Cook the eggs in a pan of boiling water for 7 mins, then rinse under cold running water to cool. Drain, peel and halve. Swirl the yogurt into the curry, then top with the eggs, chilli and coriander. Season

Red cabbage, cauliflower & coconut dhal

What You Need

1 small cauliflower, broken into small florets

2 tbsp rapeseed oil

1 onion, finely chopped

200g red cabbage, sliced

thumb-sized piece of ginger, peeled and grated

2 garlic cloves, crushed

½ tsp chilli powder

½ tsp turmeric

1 tsp garam masala

1 tsp black mustard seeds

small handful of curry leaves

300g split red lentils

1.25 litres hot low-salt vegetable stock

1 lime, juiced

2 tbsp coconut flakes, toasted

coriander leaves and chopped chilli, to serve (optional)

Directions

STEP 1

Heat the oven to 180C/160C fan/gas 4. Toss the cauliflower, 1 tbsp of the oil and some seasoning in a roasting tin. Roast for 25-30 mins, then set aside.

STEP 2

Heat the remaining oil in a large saucepan and add the onion and cabbage. Fry gently over a medium heat for 10 mins. Add the ginger, garlic, spices and curry leaves and fry for 2 mins. Stir through the lentils and most of the cauliflower. Pour over the stock, bring to the boil, lower to a simmer and cook uncovered for 40 mins. Stir through the lime juice and season to taste. Ladle into bowls, top with the remaining cauliflower, toasted coconut and coriander and chilli, if using

Carrot & ginger soup

What You Need

1 tbsp rapeseed oil

1 large onion, chopped

2 tbsp coarsely grated ginger

2 garlic cloves, sliced

½ tsp ground nutmeg

850ml vegetable stock

500g carrot (preferably organic), sliced

400g can cannellini beans (no need to drain)

Supercharged topping

4 tbsp almonds in their skins, cut into slivers

sprinkle of nutmeg

Directions

STEP 1

Heat the oil in a large pan, add the onion, ginger and garlic, and fry for 5 mins until starting to soften. Stir in the nutmeg and cook for 1 min more.

STEP 2

Pour in the stock, add the carrots, beans and their liquid, then cover and simmer for 20-25 mins until the carrots are tender.

STEP 3

Scoop a third of the mixture into a bowl and blitz the remainder with a hand blender or in a food processor until smooth. Return everything to the pan and heat until bubbling. Serve topped with the almonds and nutmeg

Sardine tomato pasta with gremolata

What You Need

75g wholemeal spaghetti

½ x 120g can sardines in oil

½ tbsp capers, drained

2 garlic cloves, crushed

2 tomatoes, roughly chopped

30g rocket

½ lemon, zested

small handful of parsley, finely chopped

Directions

STEP 1

Cook the pasta following pack instructions in a large pan of boiling salted water. Heat 1 tbsp oil from the can of sardines in a non-stick frying pan over a medium heat and sizzle the capers and half the garlic for 1-2 mins until fragrant. Tip in the tomatoes and fry for 4-5 mins more until softened and bursting. Stir in the sardines and rocket, tossing a few times to break up the fish and wilt the leaves. Season.

STEP 2

For the gremolata, combine the lemon zest, parsley and remaining garlic in a small bowl, and season. Drain the pasta and top with the sardine sauce and gremolata.

Chipotle & lime prawn burrito bowls

What You Need

1 red onion, finely sliced

2 tbsp apple cider vinegar

½ tsp caster sugar

250g leftover cooked rice

1 lime, zested and juiced, plus extra lime wedges to serve (optional)

4 spring onions, finely sliced

400g can kidney beans, drained and rinsed

198g can sweetcorn, drained

1 avocado, stoned, peeled and sliced

2 large tomatoes, finely chopped

2 tbsp low-fat crème fraîche

½ small bunch of coriander, roughly chopped

½ tsp chilli flakes (optional)

For the prawns

2 tsp chipotle paste

½ tsp honey

1 lime, zested and juiced

1 tsp olive oil

125g cooked king prawns

Directions

STEP 1

Mix the red onion with the vinegar, sugar and a pinch of salt. Cover and leave to pickle for at least 1 hr or overnight. To prepare the prawns, mix the chipotle paste, honey, lime zest and juice and oil together, then toss in the prawns until they're coated in the mixture.

STEP 2

Put the leftover rice in a large bowl and mix with the lime zest and juice, most of the spring onions and the kidney beans. Season lightly. Spoon the mixture into two shallow bowls.

STEP 3

Top the rice with the pickled red onions, spiced prawns, sweetcorn, sliced avocado, the remaining spring onions and tomatoes. Spoon the crème fraîche on top, then serve with the coriander and a sprinkling of chilli flakes, if you want it spicy. Serve the extra lime wedges on the side for squeezing over, if you like.

Roasted new potato, kale & feta salad with avocado

What You Need

200g Jersey Royal potatoes, halved

2 garlic cloves

2 tbsp cold-pressed rapeseed oil

1 lemon, juiced

1 banana shallot, chopped

200g bag kale

1 small ripe avocado, flesh scooped out

½ tsp Dijon mustard

25g feta (or vegetarian alternative), crumbled

½-1 tsp chilli flakes

1 tbsp pumpkin seeds, toasted

Directions

STEP 1

Heat oven to 200C/180C fan/gas 6. Boil the potatoes for 10 mins until mostly tender, drain and leave to steam dry. Toss the potatoes in a large roasting tin with the garlic, drizzle over 1 tbsp oil and season. Roast for 20 mins.

STEP 2

While the potatoes are roasting, squeeze half the lemon juice over the shallot and half of the kale, season, then massage gently to encourage the kale to soften.

STEP 3

Remove the garlic cloves from the oven. Put the rest of the kale on top of the potatoes, drizzle over a little oil, season and return to the oven for 5 mins until crisp.

STEP 4

Meanwhile, blitz the garlic, avocado, mustard, remaining oil and lemon juice together, add enough water to create a smooth dressing and season to taste. Mix the potatoes and cooked kale into the raw kale salad and tip onto a platter. Drizzle over the dressing, then top with the feta, chilli flakes and pumpkin seeds.

Better-than-baked beans with spicy wedges

What You Need

1 tsp oil

1 onion, halved and thinly sliced

2 rashers streaky bacon, cut into large-ish pieces

1 tsp sugar, brown if you have it

400g can chopped tomato

200ml stock from a cube

410g can cannellini bean, butter or haricot beans in water

For the wedges

1 tbsp white flour (plain or self-raising)

0.5 tsp cayenne pepper, paprika or mild chilli powder

1 tsp dried mixed herb (optional)

2 baking potatoes, each cut into 8 wedges

2 tsp oil

Directions

STEP 1

Heat oven to 200C/fan 180C/gas 6. For the wedges, mix the flour, cayenne and herbs (if using), add some salt and pepper, then toss with the potatoes and oil until well coated. Tip into a roasting tin, then bake for about 35 mins until crisp and cooked through.

STEP 2

Meanwhile, heat the oil in a non-stick pan, then gently fry the onion and bacon together for 5-10 mins until the onions are softened and just starting to turn golden. Stir in the sugar, tomatoes, stock and seasoning to taste, then simmer the sauce for 5 mins. Add the beans, then simmer for another 5 mins until the sauce has thickened. Serve with the wedges.

Roasted asparagus & pea salad

What You Need

3 tbsp natural yogurt

1 tsp wholegrain mustard

½ tsp honey

½ lemon, zested and juiced

100g watercress

1 large slice sourdough bread

200g asparagus, tough ends removed

1 ½ tbsp cold-pressed rapeseed oil

2 eggs

200g frozen peas

Directions

STEP 1

Heat oven to 220C/200C fan/gas 7. Mix the yogurt, mustard and honey together. Add the lemon zest, then add the juice and some seasoning to taste. Squeeze any remaining lemon juice over the watercress.

STEP 2

Tear the bread into rough chunks and put them on a large roasting tray with the asparagus. Toss both in the rapeseed oil and seasoning, and roast for 10 mins until the asparagus is tender and croutons are golden.

STEP 3

Meanwhile, cook the eggs in a pan of boiling water for 6 mins, then add the frozen peas and cook for 1 min more. Drain and rinse both under cold water until cool. Peel the eggs, then cut into quarters.

STEP 4

To assemble, mix the asparagus and peas through the watercress, then toss through the creamy dressing. Nestle in the eggs and croutons, and serve.

Dhal poached eggs with herby raita

What You Need

2 tbsp rapeseed oil

2 onions (320g), halved and thinly sliced

2 tsp each cumin seeds and ground turmeric

1 tsp mustard seeds

2 tbsp garam masala

4 garlic cloves, sliced

1 red chilli, deseeded and sliced

175g red lentils

400g can chickpeas

2 tsp vegetable bouillon powder, mixed with 700ml boiling water

320g baby spinach

8 large eggs

For the raita

150g natural bio yogurt

1 garlic clove

thin slice of peeled ginger

20g coriander leaves, plus a few extra leaves to serve
(optional)

10g mint leaves

Directions

STEP 1

Heat the oil in a large frying pan over a medium heat
and fry the onions for 5 mins until they start to colour.
Stir in the spices, garlic and chilli, and cook for a few
more seconds until aromatic.

STEP 2

Add the lentils, chickpeas and stock, then cook,
uncovered, for 15 mins until the lentils are tender. Stir
in the spinach until wilted.

STEP 3

Remove half the dhal from the pan and leave to cool. Will keep chilled for up to three days. Break 4 eggs, spaced apart, into the lentils that are left in the pan, cover and cook over a medium heat for 8-10 mins.

STEP 4

Meanwhile, put all the What You Need for the raita in a bowl and blitz together using a hand blender.

STEP 5

Serve the eggs and dhal with half the raita and scatter over a few extra coriander leaves, if you like. The remaining raita will keep chilled for up to three days. Reheat the remaining dhal in a pan over a medium heat until bubbling. Add a drop of water if it looks dry, then cook the eggs in the hot dhal as described in step 3 and serve with the remaining raita.

Spinach falafel & hummus bowl

What You Need

150g baby spinach

½ cucumber, sliced

1 red onion, finely sliced

4 wholemeal pittas, toasted, to serve

For the falafel

150g baby spinach

400g can chickpeas, drained

1 garlic clove, chopped

1 tsp ground cumin

½ small bunch of parsley, finely chopped

2 tbsp plain flour

1 tbsp olive oil, plus extra for rolling

For the hummus

400g chickpeas, drained

40ml olive oil, plus extra to serve

1 garlic clove, roughly chopped

1 lemon, juiced, plus extra to serve (optional)

2 tbsp tahini

Directions

STEP 1

Heat the oven to 190C/170C fan/gas 5. Line a baking sheet with non-stick parchment. Put all the falafel What You Need, except for the oil, in a food processor and season lightly. Pulse until you have a rough mix.

STEP 2

Oil your hands lightly, then take tablespoons of the falafel mix, roll into around 16 balls and put on the baking sheet. Press each one down slightly with the palm of your hand. Brush using the 1 tbsp oil and bake for 20-25 mins until firm and golden, turning halfway through.

STEP 3

While the falafel is cooking, make the hummus. Put all of the hummus *What You Need* into a food processor with 50ml of water and blitz until smooth and silky.

STEP 4

Put the spinach, cucumber, red onion and falafel in different sections of each bowl, alongside some hummus, then drizzle with the extra olive oil. Grind over some black pepper. Serve with the pittas on the side and more lemon for squeezing over, if you like.

Egg-fried noodles with beansprouts

What You Need

2 dried wholemeal noodle nests (about 100g)

2 limes, juiced

1 tsp tamari

2 garlic cloves, 1 finely grated, 1 chopped

1 red chilli, deseeded and finely sliced

1 tbsp sesame or rapeseed oil

2 red onions, (200g), halved and thinly sliced

15g ginger, peeled and cut into fine shreds

1 small red pepper, deseeded and cut into strips

1 tbsp medium curry powder

200g ready-to-eat beansprouts, rinsed and drained

1 tbsp tahini

3 eggs, beaten

15g coriander, chopped

Directions

STEP 1

Cook the noodles following pack instructions. Combine the lime juice, tamari, grated garlic and chilli in a small bowl. Set aside.

STEP 2

Heat the oil in a non-stick wok or large, wide pan over a high heat and stir-fry the onions, ginger and pepper for 5 mins until softened (add the chopped garlic for the last minute). Stir in the curry powder and cook for a minute more. Add the beansprouts and continue cooking until the beansprouts start to soften and are piping hot. Mix in the tahini.

STEP 3

Push the veg to the side of the wok and pour in the egg – you may need a drop more oil. Stir-fry the eggs so they are mostly set, then stir the veg into the egg and add the noodles and coriander, then toss to combine. Pile into bowls and serve with the sauce on the side

Caponata with cheesy polenta

What You Need

1-2 tbsp olive oil

1 red onion, cut into thin wedges

1 courgette, cut into rounds

1 aubergine, cut into chunks

2 garlic cloves, crushed

2 tsp dried oregano

¼ tsp chilli flakes

400g can chopped tomatoes

30g pitted green olives, halved

½ tbsp capers, drained and rinsed

½ small bunch of basil, finely chopped, plus extra to serve

100g instant polenta

a little milk, to loosen (optional)

40g parmesan or vegetarian Italian-style hard cheese, grated

Directions

STEP 1

Heat the oil in a medium pan set over a medium heat, and fry the onion, courgette and aubergine for 5-10 mins, or until beginning to soften. Stir in the garlic, oregano and chilli flakes, followed by the tomatoes, olives and capers. Season to taste, then simmer, covered, for 20 mins, or until all the veg is soft and cooked through. Stir in the basil and taste for seasoning.

STEP 2

Meanwhile, cook the polenta following pack instructions – you may need to loosen with some water or milk if it's too thick. Mix with the parmesan, then spoon and spread over two plates. Top with the caponata and extra basil. Season.

Miso roast salmon, lentil & pomegranate salad

What You Need

80g dried puy lentils

1 tsp miso paste

2 tsp finely grated ginger

1 garlic clove, finely grated

1 lime, zested and juiced

1 tsp olive oil

½ tsp black/white sesame seeds

2 x 150g skinless wild salmon fillets

1 tsp apple cider vinegar

2 carrots, cut into fine strips with a julienne peeler or knife

60g pomegranate seeds

3 spring onions, finely sliced

handful fresh coriander, chopped

Directions

STEP 1

Heat oven to 200C/180C fan/gas 6. Cook the lentils in a pan of boiling water for 20 mins until tender. Meanwhile, mix the miso paste with 1 tsp of the ginger, the garlic, half the lime juice, the oil and sesame seeds. Put the salmon fillets on a foil-lined baking tray and spread 1 tbsp of the miso mixture over them. Roast for 10-12 mins until cooked through.

STEP 2

Tip the rest of the miso mixture into a bowl with the remaining ginger and lime juice. Add the lime zest, vinegar, carrots, pomegranate, onions and coriander. Drain the lentils and toss into the salad. Divide between two plates and add the salmon.

Healthy seafood pasta recipe

What You Need

2 tbsp olive or rapeseed oil

1 small fennel bulb (160g), halved and thinly sliced

1 onion (160g), finely chopped

150g wholemeal spaghetti

2 large pinches of chilli flakes

3 garlic cloves, finely grated

½ lemon, zested, plus 2 tbsp juice

3 tbsp tomato purée

300g frozen mixed seafood (we used a mixture of prawns, mussels and squid rings), defrosted

3 tbsp chopped parsley

Directions

STEP 1

Heat the oil in a large non-stick pan and cook the fennel and onion for 10 mins, stirring occasionally until softened. Meanwhile, bring a pan of water to the boil and cook the spaghetti for 10 mins until al dente.

STEP 2

When the fennel and onion mixture has softened, stir in the chilli flakes, garlic, lemon zest and juice. Add the tomato purée and cook briefly, stirring all the time.

STEP 3

Drain the pasta, reserving a mugful (around 250ml) of the cooking water. Stir the seafood into the tomato sauce and warm through. Toss the spaghetti into the sauce with the parsley and just enough of the reserved cooking water to loosen. Season and serve.

Chorizo & chickpea summer stew

What You Need

1 tbsp olive oil

2 garlic cloves, crushed

2 thyme sprigs

1 tbsp smoked paprika

200g chorizo ring, sliced into thin coins

1 tbsp sherry vinegar

600g cherry tomatoes, halved

450g jar roasted red peppers, drained and cut into large strips

100g spinach

2 x 400g cans chickpeas, drained

drizzle of extra virgin olive oil and crusty bread, to serve

Directions

STEP 1

Heat the oil in a large frying pan over a medium heat, add the garlic, thyme and smoked paprika, and stir for a few minutes, then tip in the chorizo and stir for another couple of minutes until its oil is released. Splash in the sherry vinegar and let it bubble for a minute or so.

STEP 2

Add the tomatoes, peppers, spinach and chickpeas along with 100ml water and a pinch of seasoning. Bring to the boil, then reduce the heat to a simmer and cook until the tomatoes have softened and there is a thickened sauce, about 15 mins. Adjust the seasoning and finish with a drizzle of extra virgin olive oil. Serve with crusty bread

Vegan roast spiced squash salad with tahini dressing

What You Need

320g diced butternut squash

3 red onions (320g), cut into wedges

2 tbsp rapeseed oil

2 tsp smoked paprika

1 tsp cumin seeds

2 tbsp chopped thyme

125g quinoa

½ x 85g bag kale

2 tbsp pumpkin seeds

2 tbsp tahini

2 tbsp apple cider vinegar

1 garlic clove, finely grated

2 x 400g cans lentils or borlotti beans, very well drained

50g pomegranate seeds

4 generous handfuls of rocket

Directions

STEP 1

Heat the oven to 200C/180C fan/gas 6. Tip the squash and onions onto a large baking sheet and toss with 1 tsp of the oil. Spread out and sprinkle with the paprika, cumin and thyme, then roast for 30 mins.

STEP 2

Meanwhile, cook the quinoa following pack instructions, then drain well (or the base of the salad will be too wet).

STEP 3

Add the kale to the tray of veg, sprinkle over the seeds and return to the oven for 10 mins.

STEP 4

For the dressing, mix the tahini and remaining oil with the vinegar, garlic and 2 tbsp water.

STEP 5

Put the quinoa in a bowl and toss with the lentils or beans. Pile half into a salad bowl and the rest into two lunchboxes or bowls, if you're following the Healthy Diet Plan. Divide the veg on top, then drizzle with the dressing, scatter over the pomegranate seeds and top with the rocket. Chill the other two portions for the next day. Will keep chilled for up to three days.

Minty griddled chicken & peach salad

What You Need

1 lime, zested and juiced

1 tbsp rapeseed oil

2 tbsp mint, finely chopped, plus a few leaves to serve

1 garlic clove, finely grated

2 skinless chicken breast fillets (300g)

160g fine beans, trimmed and halved

2 peaches (200g), each cut into 8 thick wedges

1 red onion, cut into wedges

1 large Little Gem lettuce (165g), roughly shredded

½ x 60g pack rocket

1 small avocado, stoned and sliced

240g cooked new potatoes

Directions

STEP 1

Mix the lime zest and juice, oil and mint, then put half in a bowl with the garlic. Thickly slice the chicken at a slight angle, add to the garlic mixture and toss together with plenty of black pepper.

STEP 2

Cook the beans in a pan of water for 3-4 mins until just tender. Meanwhile, griddle the chicken and onion for a few mins each side until cooked and tender. Transfer to a plate, then quickly griddle the peaches. If you don't have a griddle pan, use a non-stick frying pan with a drop of oil.

STEP 3

Toss the warm beans and onion in the remaining mint mixture, and pile onto a platter or into individual shallow bowls with the lettuce and rocket. Top with the avocado, peaches and chicken and scatter over the mint. Serve with the potatoes while still warm.

Pasta with chilli tomatoes & spinach

What You Need

2 tsp olive oil

1 onion, finely chopped

2 garlic cloves, crushed

½ tsp dried chilli flakes

200g wholemeal penne pasta

400g can chopped tomato

100ml red wine

½ tsp dried oregano

125g bag young spinach leaves

25g parmesan or vegetarian alternative, grated

Directions

STEP 1

Heat the oil in a non-stick frying pan and gently fry the onion, garlic and chilli flakes, stirring regularly, for 5 mins (add a little water if they begin to stick).

STEP 2

Cook pasta following pack instructions. Add the tomatoes, wine and oregano to the frying pan and stir to combine. Bring to a gentle simmer and cook, stirring occasionally, for 10 mins.

STEP 3

Shake the spinach into the pan and cook for 1-2 mins until wilted. Drain the pasta and tip into the pan with the sauce. Toss to combine, sprinkle with cheese and serve.

Super-green mac 'n' cheese

What You Need

1l semi-skimmed milk

75g butter

75g plain flour

2 tsp Dijon mustard

175g mature or extra mature cheddar, grated

50g parmesan, grated

100g spinach, fresh or frozen

400g macaroni

1 broccoli (about 300g), broken into florets

100g frozen peas

For the topping (optional)

3 slices white bread (about 125g)

1 small bunch of basil leaves

1 tsp olive oil

25g mixed nuts or seeds, such as pumpkin seeds, pine nuts and almonds, for the topping

Directions

STEP 1

Heat the oven to 220C/200C fan/gas 7. Tip the milk, butter and flour into a large saucepan and bring to a simmer, whisking continuously until you have a smooth, thick sauce, about 3-4 mins. Don't worry if there are a few lumps – the sauce will be blended later. Season well, then add the mustard, both cheeses and spinach.

STEP 2

Meanwhile, cook the pasta in boiling salted water for 5 mins. Add the broccoli and continue cooking until the pasta is cooked through and the broccoli is soft. Drain.

STEP 3

Transfer half the cooked broccoli to the cheese sauce. Whizz the cheese sauce until smooth, creamy and bright green using a hand blender (or stand mixer). Loosen with a splash of milk, if needed. Stir in the pasta, remaining broccoli and the peas and tip into a large baking dish.

STEP 4

If making the topping, put the bread, basil, oil and half the nuts or seeds in a food processor and whizz to coarse, green crumbs. Scatter over the pasta along with the remaining nuts or seeds. Bake for 20-25 mins, until the topping is crunchy and the sauce is bubbling. Will keep in an airtight container in the freezer for up to three months.

Pork with cucumber & apricot couscous

What You Need

30g fresh coriander

4 small garlic cloves, chopped

2 tsp sumac

1 tbsp olive oil

400g pork fillet

1½ tsp smoked paprika

For the couscous

drop of olive oil, for roasting

2 red onions, halved and sliced

1 aubergine, cut into 1cm cubes

200g wholemeal giant couscous

small bunch of spring onions (about 100g), sliced

½ large cucumber (about 320g), chopped

1 lemon, zested plus 2 tbsp juice

2 tbsp extra virgin olive oil

15g mint, leaves chopped

8 fresh apricots (about 320g)

25g toasted flaked almonds

Directions

STEP 1

Heat the oven to 190C/170C fan/gas 5. Put the coriander in a small bowl with the garlic, sumac, oil and 2 tbsp water, then blitz using a hand blender until smooth. Rub a quarter of it all over the pork, then put the pork on a large baking tray and sprinkle over the paprika.

STEP 2

For the couscous, rub a drop of oil over the red onions and aubergine, then scatter around the pork. (If your tray isn't large enough, use two.) Roast for 25 mins. Check the pork and if it isn't cooked but the vegetables are, take the vegetables out of the oven and cook the pork for another 10-15 mins until the juices run clear.

STEP 3

Meanwhile, cook the couscous following pack instructions, then drain and tip into a bowl with the remaining garlicky herb mixture. Add the spring onions, cucumber, lemon zest and juice, extra virgin olive oil and mint. Quarter and stone the apricots. If ripe, add the apricots to the salad bowl, but if a little firm, add them to the tray in the oven first to cook for 10 mins until softened.

STEP 4

Set the pork aside to rest. Add the roasted red onions, aubergine, apricots and almonds to the couscous and toss everything together. Slice the pork, serve half with half the couscous, and chill the rest for another day to eat cold.

Will keep chilled for two to three days.

Mexican salmon salad

What You Need

2 tortillas

2 tbsp olive oil

½ tsp ground coriander

3 tbsp Greek yogurt

1 tsp smoked paprika

2 salmon fillets

1 lime, zested and juiced

2 Little Gem lettuces, separated into leaves

198g can sweetcorn, drained

½small pack coriander, roughly chopped

300g pack cherry tomatoes, halved

Directions

STEP 1

Heat oven to 200C/fan 180C/gas 6. Cut the tortillas into triangles using scissors, toss in 1 tbsp of the oil and the ground coriander, season, then tip onto a lined baking sheet. Bake for 8-10 mins, turning halfway, until crisp. Set aside to cool. Heat the grill to high.

STEP 2

Mix the yogurt with the smoked paprika and some seasoning, then spoon the yogurt mixture over the salmon. Place fillets on the same baking sheet, lined with parchment, and put under the grill for 8-10 mins until the fish is blackening in places, and flakes into big chunks.

STEP 3

While the salmon is cooking, whisk the remaining olive oil with the lime zest and juice to make a dressing, season, then toss the remaining salad **What You Need** in the dressing. Tip onto a plate, top with the salmon chunks and tortilla chips and serve.

Beetroot & feta pasta

What You Need

2 large beetroots, peeled and roughly chopped into chunks

1 tbsp olive oil

2 onions, finely chopped

4 celery sticks, finely chopped, celery tops kept separate

4 carrots, peeled and finely chopped

1 small bunch of basil

2 garlic cloves, finely chopped

400g wholemeal pasta

75g low-fat crème fraîche

100g feta

Directions

STEP 1

Put a large pan of salted water on a high heat, bring to the boil and add the beetroot chunks. Boil for 5 mins, then transfer the beetroot to a plate using a slotted spoon. Set the pan of cooking water aside.

STEP 2

Meanwhile, put the olive oil in a large frying pan set over a medium heat, then add the onions, celery and carrots, and cook for 8 mins until softened. Finely chop the basil stalks and celery tops, then add to the pan along with the garlic, and fry for another 30 seconds.

STEP 3

Tip the pasta into the pan of beetroot water and simmer for 13-15 mins (depending on what pasta you're using) until just cooked but retaining a little bite. Drain, reserving 200ml of the pasta water and tip the pasta back into the pan.

STEP 4

Meanwhile, put the beetroot with half of the fried veg into the bowl of a food processor with most of the basil leaves and the crème fraîche, then blitz until smooth. Gradually add the reserved pasta water to loosen until you have a thick mixture.

STEP 5

Stir this sauce through the pasta along with the remaining fried veg and some seasoning. Divide between bowls, crumble over the feta, then scatter with the remaining basil leaves. Grind over some black pepper, if you like

Lemon & spinach rice with feta

What You Need

1 tbsp rapeseed oil

2 onions (320g), finely chopped

3 large garlic cloves, sliced

300g easy-cook brown rice

700ml hot vegetable stock, made with 1 tsp bouillon powder

400g frozen spinach

15g dill, finely chopped

1 lemon, zested, 1/2 juiced, 1/2 cut into 4 wedges

40g walnuts, chopped

75g feta, crumbled

Directions

STEP 1

Heat the oil in a large pan over a medium heat and fry the onions and garlic for 10 mins, stirring often until softened.

STEP 2

Tip in the rice, then the stock, frozen spinach and half each of the dill and lemon zest. Cover, reduce the heat to low and cook for 25 mins until the rice is tender.

STEP 3

Scatter over the remaining dill and lemon zest, the nuts and feta, then gently toss together along with the lemon juice. Serve half of the rice straightaway with two lemon wedges on the side for squeezing over. Leave the rest of the rice to cool completely and keep chilled for up to three days. Reheat in the microwave until piping hot, then serve with the remaining lemon wedges.

This recipe is part of our free 7-day healthy diet plan. This easy-to-follow, nutritionist-created plan will inspire you to cook and eat more healthily. Nourish yourself with seven days of meals, snacks and treats.

Curried spinach & lentil soup

What You Need

2 tbsp rapeseed oil

1 onion, finely chopped

2 large garlic cloves, crushed

¼ tsp hot chilli powder

1 tsp cumin seeds

1 tbsp medium curry powder

160g dried brown lentils

1.2l low-salt veg stock

large bunch coriander

30g unsalted cashew nuts, toasted

2 lemons, zested and juiced

500g spinach

Directions

STEP 1

Heat 1 tbsp oil in a large saucepan. Add the onion and fry for 8 mins until soft and translucent. Stir in half the garlic, the chilli, cumin and curry powder and cook for 1 min more. Add the lentils and stock, then cover and simmer for 30 mins over a medium-low heat.

STEP 2

Put the coriander, remaining oil and garlic, the cashews and lemon zest in a food processor and blitz with 1-2 tbsp water until semi-smooth. Spoon the chutney into a bowl and set aside.

STEP 3

Stir the spinach into the soup and cook for 5 mins, or until wilted. Tip half the soup into a blender and blitz until smooth, then return this to the pan. Stir through lemon juice to taste.

STEP 4

Ladle the soup into bowls and top with generous dollops of the cashew chutney.

Tomato & mascarpone risotto

What You Need

2 tbsp olive oil

1 onion, very finely chopped

1 large garlic clove, crushed

175g risotto rice

400g can cherry tomatoes

600ml hot vegetable stock

30g parmesan or vegetarian alternative, grated

30g mascarpone, or cream cheese

½ small bunch of basil, chopped

Directions

STEP 1

Heat the oil in a large, heavy-based saucepan. Add the onion along with a pinch of salt, and fry for 10 mins or until beginning to soften and turn translucent, then add the garlic and fry for 1 min. Stir in the rice and cook for 2 mins.

STEP 2

Tip in the tomatoes and bring to a simmer. Add half the stock, cooking and stirring until absorbed. Add the remaining stock, a ladleful at a time, and cook until the rice is al dente, stirring constantly for around 20 mins.

STEP 3

Stir through the parmesan, mascarpone or cream cheese, and basil, then season to taste. Spoon into bowls to serve

Vegetarian bean pot with herby breadcrumbs

What You Need

1 slice crusty bread

½ small pack parsley leaves

½ lemon, zested

2 tbsp olive oil

pinch chilli flakes (optional)

2 leeks, rinsed and chopped into half-moons

2 carrots, thinly sliced

2 celery sticks, thinly sliced

1 fennel bulb, thinly sliced

2 large garlic cloves, chopped

1 tbsp tomato purée

few thyme sprigs

150ml white wine

400g can cannellini beans, drained

Directions

STEP 1

Toast the bread, then tear into pieces and put in a food processor with the parsley, lemon zest, ½ tbsp olive oil, a good pinch of salt and pepper and the chilli flakes, if using. Blitz to breadcrumbs. Set aside.

STEP 2

Heat the remaining oil in a pan and add the leeks, carrots, celery and fennel along with a splash of water and a pinch of salt. Cook over a medium heat for 10 mins until soft, then add the garlic and tomato purée. Cook for 1 min more, then add the thyme and white wine. Leave to bubble for a minute, then add the beans. Fill the can halfway with water and pour into the pot.

STEP 3

Bring the cassoulet to the boil, then turn down the heat and leave to simmer for 15 mins before removing the thyme sprigs. Mash half the beans to thicken the stew. Season to taste, then divide between bowls and top with the herby breadcrumbs to serve.

SECTION 7: IN SUMMARY

In conclusion, the Circadian Diet represents a multifaceted approach to not only weight management but also holistic health and well-being. Throughout the pages of this book, we've explored the intricate interplay between our dietary habits and our body's internal clock, shedding light on the profound impact that timing and nutrient composition can have on our physiology.

At its core, the Circadian Diet is rooted in the fundamental principle of synchronizing our eating patterns with our circadian rhythms, the innate biological processes that regulate our sleep-wake cycle, metabolism, and numerous other bodily functions. By honoring these natural rhythms and aligning our meals accordingly, we can harness the power of our biology to optimize digestion, metabolism, and energy utilization.

One of the key tenets of the Circadian Diet is the concept of time-restricted eating, which involves confining our daily food intake to a specific window of time, typically aligned with daylight hours. This practice not only enhances metabolic efficiency but also promotes better sleep quality and overall health. By allowing our bodies ample time to digest and metabolize food before the onset of restorative sleep, we support the body's natural detoxification and repair processes, leading to improved health outcomes.

Furthermore, the Circadian Diet emphasizes the importance of nutrient timing, encouraging individuals to consume larger meals earlier in the day when metabolic activity is highest and tapering off food intake in the evening when the body's energy demands diminish. This approach not only optimizes nutrient absorption and utilization but also helps regulate appetite and reduce the risk of overeating, particularly during nighttime hours when metabolic function is naturally lower.

Beyond timing, the Circadian Diet places a strong emphasis on the quality of food choices, advocating for a balanced and nutrient-dense diet rich in whole, unprocessed foods. By prioritizing fresh fruits and vegetables, lean proteins, healthy fats, and whole grains, we provide our bodies with the essential nutrients needed to support optimal health and vitality. Moreover, by minimizing the consumption of processed foods, refined sugars, and artificial additives, we reduce the risk of chronic disease and promote longevity.

As we've explored the principles and practical applications of the Circadian Diet, it's evident that this dietary approach offers a comprehensive framework for achieving and maintaining optimal health. By embracing the wisdom of our body's internal clock and aligning our eating patterns with the rhythms of nature, we can unlock our full potential for vitality and well-being. However, it's important to recognize that the Circadian Diet is not a one-size-fits-all solution and may need to be tailored to individual needs and preferences.

In the quest for optimal health and wellness, the Circadian Diet stands as a beacon of hope, offering a scientifically grounded approach to nourishing our bodies and supporting our overall well-being. With further research and practical application, this dietary paradigm has the potential to transform the way we think about food and health, paving the way for a brighter, healthier future for generations to come.